KETO COOBOOK FOR WOMEN OVER 50

The Ultimate Keto Diet Guide For Senior Women.

A Cookbook That Includes 90+ Delicious Keto Recipes For Healthy Weight Loss. Reset Your Metabolism And Boost Energy.

BY

PATRICIA VOGEL

Table Of Contents

WHY THIS BOOK?

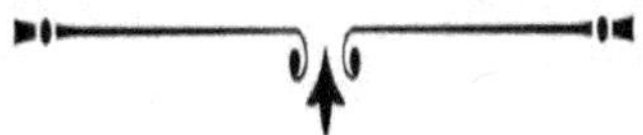

Keeping the body fit and healthy when a woman goes beyond the golden jubilee landmark is almost an impossible task. However, like the famous saying goes 'nothing is impossible', you must have come across some over 50 ladies who look 20 and are almost or even healthier than some ladies in their 20's. Do you know you can also live a healthy life and have a fit body when you are past 50? This is what KETO diet provides for a woman and that is what this book is all about.

The first chapter focuses on the basics about ketogenic diets, how they work in the body, what ketosis is all about and how to understand the dynamics around it and how the diet works for women above 50.

The second chapter delves deeply into the general benefit of sticking with keto diets and even more specifically on how women above 50 can have fitness they so much desire and live healthily.

There is no good thing in the world that doesn't come with its own unique challenges and keto diet is no different. There are some challenges peculiar to keto diet with people of different age grade and sex. Chapter three of the book focuses on the possible challenges that women may face from the consumption of keto diet and how they can void these so-called challenges.

The next chapter focuses on the nutritional composition of keto diets generally and the types of food which can be used for the diet.

The final chapter takes a gander at different types of keto diet recipes with clear and concise instructions on the ingredients, how to cook them and the nutritional composition of each of them.

KETO 101

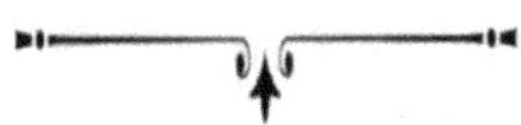

INTRODUCTION

Have you at any point needed to have more vitality in your day, feel much improved and look better? Numerous individuals have figured out how to accomplish a superior existence with a straightforward diet. I know it sounds unrealistic. However, it is extremely conceivable to acquire vitality, feel much improved and look better by changing how you eat. There is no enchantment pill; rather it is as straightforward as building up an eating plan that gives your body the supplements it needs.

The ketogenic diet, also called the keto diet, is anything but a novel trend diet dependent on insecure dietary science. It has been around since the past times, with antiquated Greeks using the diet as a feature of an all-encompassing treatment for epilepsy. Truth be told, here in the States, it was a recognized method for treatment for youth epileptic seizures all through the 1920s. Lamentably, this regular method for treatment needed to offer a route to the cutting edge advances of pharmaceutical science with its affinity for quick impacts. Joyfully, the ketogenic diet has discovered its way again into the standard yet again and likely for excellent reasons! The premise of the diet is to basically trigger your body's own fat consuming components to fuel what the body requires for vitality for the day. This implies the fat that you eat, just as the put-away fat in your body, have all become fuel stores your body can tap on! Little marvel that this diet truly causes you with weight reduction, in any event, for those difficult, difficult to lose greasy territories. That could be one reason why you picked this book and investigated leaving on the ketogenic excursion, or you may have heard stuff from your group of friends about how the keto diet really standardizes glucose levels just as enhances your cholesterol readings and you are fascinated. What about stories of type 2 diabetes being turned around simply through after this diet alone, as well as stories of specific malignancies being ended or the tumors contracting due to the constructive outcomes of the keto diet? We should likewise not overlook the going with a chance decrease of cardiovascular sickness because of the diet!

The entirety of the advantages referenced above stem to a great extent from a solitary significant process in the ketogenic diet. Ketosis is the name of the game. A Ketogenic Diet is any diet that makes ketones be created by the liver, moving the body's digestion away from glucose towards fat usage. Regularly on a moderate to high carb diet, the body will lean toward glucose for fuel (generally from dietary carbs), yet by confining carbs, the body will incline toward fat for fuel. By prompting ketosis, a progression of adjustments will happen. Ketosis is, likewise a successful method to control your glucose. At the point when you eat something high in sugars, your body produces insulin to dispose of all the sugar in your blood. Be that as it may, since there is as of now carbs to be utilized for fuel, your body will store fat cells and not discharging any to be copied. So by diminishing carbs and being in ketosis, your insulin levels will be directed at a lower level; furthermore, your body will need to get to your muscle versus fat for fuel. By and large, this implies noteworthy weight reduction! With controlled glucose levels, you will encounter less yearning and desires. Combined with a sufficient protein and high fat admission, you will feel both fulfilled and satisfied by the diet.

What do I eat?

An ordinary Ketogenic Diet is any diet which confines starches between 0- 50g of carbs every day. The general proposal of keto is, to begin with 20g of net carbs every day. This utmost works admirably of taking out shoddy nourishments, refined sugars and some other "stuffing" nourishments. Net-carbs are the absolute carbs short the fiber carbs (fiber doesn't tally in light of the fact that your body doesn't assimilate it). For instance, a cup of slashed broccoli is

6g of absolute carbs and 2g of fiber. 6g - 2g = 4g net carbs. Your carbs should undeniably originate from entire nourishment sources, for example, vegetables, nuts, dairy, and so on. Attempt your best to keep away from refined starches, for example, bread, pasta, and grains; starches, for example, potatoes, beans and vegetables; and other refined sugars, for example, white sugar, HFCS, and even sugar from natural products.

Most dinners should concentrate on a protein and fat with a side of vegetables. A few models would be; a steak with a side of sautéed spinach, or chicken thighs with a side of broccoli and cheddar sauce. Tidbits can incorporate nuts and seeds, cheddar, or anything "ketoaccommodating". If all else fails, check the sustenance mark or google the carb tally to check whether it fits inside your day by day carb objective.

Side note: Be careful about cases, for example, 'powerful carbs' or 'net carbs'. A considerable lot of these things will utilize sugar alcohols, which do in-truth tally (in any event in part) and will affect your glucose. Satisfactory protein is likewise a significant part of the Ketogenic Diet and it will assist you with saving bulk.

What segment of fat/protein/carbs do I need?

One of the mantras of low-carb diets is the proportion of macronutrients "60/35/5". This implies the level of your everyday caloric admission should be sixty percent from fat, thirty-five from protein and five from starches. Fat and protein keep you full, so a greater amount of them is frequently wanted to normally keep you in a calorie shortage. Even though macronutrient proportions are a decent beginning stage, they aren't constantly precise. Another strategy is to pick a carb objective between 15-50g/day (20g is a decent beginning stage), set your protein necessities (1.5-1.75g of protein per kilogram of perfect body weight), and fill the remainder of your calories with fat.

Do I have to check calories?

Much of the time, a Ketogenic Diet will assist you with decreasing your caloric admission normally. A few people don't check calories while others do, it's actually an individual choice! Be that as it may, in the event that you aren't checking calories and you discover your weight reduction is slowing down, at that point think about following.

What happens when my body adjusts?

As you adjust to ketosis, your body will start to drain its glycogen stores. Your body is typically prepared to utilize this modest, quick and simple to-process vitality source, and it needs some an opportunity to become accustomed to running off fat as its essential wellspring of fuel. To be obtuse, you may feel like poop while adjusting. You may encounter queasiness, migraines, dazedness, mental haze, and other influenza-like manifestations. This marvel is frequently called 'keto-influenza' or 'carb-influenza. Ordinarily, this is the consequence of your electrolytes being flushed out alongside water weight.

On the off chance that you drink some conventional chicken or hamburger soup, you can renew your electrolytes and facilitate your side effects. It is likewise unbelievably essential to drink a lot of water! Your water admission will keep you hydrated and it will help flush out overabundance ketones.

Fun truth: The body can discharge up to 100 calories worth of ketones every day. This absolute adjustment process takes around three weeks to occur. During this time, you might be proceeding with an activity routine or you may even be beginning another one. You may find that you don't have as a lot of perseverance and quality as you are utilized to, and this is typical. When you are completely ketoadjusted, your body will be prepared to work on fat as its essential wellspring of fuel, and you will see an improvement in your vitality levels. Many even report having more vitality, and progressively steady vitality levels while in ketosis.

Ketosis Know How (Overview)

Ketosis is a state made by the liver. Intended to give vitality to organs and the cells, it Can supplant glucose. In our traditional Carbohydrate-rich diet, we get most of our vitality from glucose, which is converted from the carbs that we eat during dinners.

Glucose is a source that is speedy of vitality, where insulin is expected to fire up and permit glucose to stream it very well may be used as fuel for the Mitochondria alluded to as the vitality processing plants inside our cells. The more starches we ingest, the more sugar will be inside our blood, which implies the pancreas should create more insulin all together to facilitate vitality generation from the accessible blood glucose. In a body where the work is typical, the insulin is acknowledged by blood glucose as vitality.

The issue is that our cells may really become Insulin desensitized, prompting a situation where the pancreas is constrained to pump increasingly more insulin standardize and to clear the blood glucose levels. Insulin de-affectability or insulin obstruction is made for the most part due to persistent raised presence of glucose in the circulatory system Ingestion of nourishments.

Think about your body's cells as a bouncer in a club, where the passage to the club necessitates that you pay an expense. Glucose here, and furthermore is insulin. On the off chance that your frequency into the club is reliable with the standard, the bouncer doesn't recognize anything uncommon thus doesn't build the charge required for passage. Be that as it may if you show up only your urgent want and lifts the insulin charge to let the sugar. The extra charge gets ever more elevated until Where the root is the pancreas, no a spot Longer produces any. This is the place the situation will most likely be distinguished as type 2. The arrangement and diabetes would involve being on a lifetime of medications or insulin shots. The essence of the issue here lies within sight of glucose framework.

Each time we take a supper, which isn't hard right now time of cheap food and sugary treats, our glucose levels get raised, and insulin is enacted for the change. This is the place the chaos that is typical emerges, with condemnations coming in for glucose and insulin similar to the root of Many maladies and feared weight gain. I might want to take this opportunity to express that insulin and glucose are certainly not the beginning of all underhanded, as some books have portrayed them. It'd be undeniably progressively precise to arrange. To like the reason for weight and metabolic our flow day by day diet diseases tormenting the piece of the created world. Cue. The keto diet is a fat-based diet, with attention on being glaringly low carb.

This strategy is planned with the goal that we decrease our admission of sugary and Starchy nourishments that are advantageously advertised. An enjoyment actuality: glucose used as an additive in the occasions, and it's no happenstance that Much of the handled nourishments today, we as a whole contain elevated levels of sugar just because it takes into consideration a period of usability that is stretched.

Nourishments high in sugar additionally have Been demonstrated to actuate the craving response in the mind, essentially Causing one to eat for delight rather than hunger that is genuine. Studies Have uncovered that sugary treats are associated with the districts of the cerebrum that are Additionally liable for betting and medication reliance. Presently you comprehend why you can not appear to stop popping those confections into your mouth! So we cut down on the carbs, and this is the place fats are in to supplant the Energy required to continue the whole body.

Here is a portion of the numerous medical advantages that originate from being in ketosis:

- Normal yearning and craving control
- Easy weight reduction and support
- Mental lucidity
- Sounder, increasingly serene rest
- Standardized metabolic capacity
- Balanced out glucose and reestablished insulin affectability

- Lower irritation levels
- Sentiments of satisfaction and general prosperity
- Brought down circulatory strain
- Expanded HDL (great) cholesterol
- Diminished triglycerides
- Brought down or dispensed with little LDL particles (terrible cholesterol)
- Capacity to go twelve to twenty-four hours between suppers
- Utilization of put away muscle to fat ratio as a fuel source
- Unending vitality
- Dispensed with heartburn Better ripeness
- Counteraction of horrendous mind damage
- Expanded sex drive
- Improved safe framework
- Eased back maturing because of the decrease in free extreme creation
- Enhancements in blood science
- Advanced psychological capacity and improved memory
- Decreased skin inflammation breakouts and other skin conditions
- Elevated comprehension of how nourishments influence your body
- Enhancements in metabolic wellbeing markers
- Quicker and better recuperation from work out ☐ Diminished tension and emotional episodes

I could continue forever; however I think you get the thought. Ketosis is something you might need to seek after in the event that you are managing weight or medical problems and you're not getting the outcomes you want with your present technique. Later on in the book, we will examine different wellbeing conditions that are significantly improved by a ketogenic diet, reacting stunningly better to it than to probably the best prescriptions accessible. It's energizing to imagine that you could see such stunning improvement utilizing sustenance as opposed to medication.

On the ketogenic diet, you might be hoping to take in 75% of your calories as sugars Proteins and the staying 5 percent in the sort of starches. We do this since You recall that we need fats to turn into our wellspring of fuel. Only With the blend of chopping carbs down and raising our utilization will We trigger the body to start ketosis. If we do it through the diet which empowers long haul and supportable use, or we starve ourselves to ketosis. That's right, you heard me, ketosis is your body reason That gathers a cradle against those occasions when nourishment is rare.

HOW DO I GUARANTEE I'M IN KETOSIS?

A simple method to know without a doubt you are in ketosis is to utilize ketosis. These little sticks can be found in many drug stores and even on the web. They test for abundance ketones, so they aren't generally the most dependable, yet in the event that you see a positive on the stick, you are destined to be in ketosis. Different indications of ketosis may be; an amusing preference for your mouth, your pee will smell extraordinary or you're unfathomably parched. Be that as it may, on the off chance that you have been eating 20g of carbs a day for at any rate 3 days, you are more than likely in ketosis.

I DON'T THINK I CAN GIVE UP CARBS!

When you overcome the underlying challenge of carb longings, they leave! Since keto will balance out your glucose, it will likewise balance out your appetite and longings. Since your body is presently changing following a low-sugar diet, you will find that your taste buds will change too and you can now effectively distinguish the sugar content in certain nourishments. Things, for example, carrots and dull chocolate currently taste better. The longer you stick to keto and the stricter you are, the less you will miss carbs. Carbs and sugar are really addictive, and like any other person attempting to break enslavement, the best technique is to remove the wellspring of the issue.

HOW THE BODY REACTS TO KETO FOODS

There are two accessible wellsprings of fuel for the human body: sugar (glucose) and fat. Ketones are delivered when the body consumes fat, and these are what power modules. The objective of the ketogenic diet is to get the body to use fat as opposed to sugar. Being a fat killer is called being keto-adjusted, and it is the liked metabolic condition of the human body. It generally takes two to about a month on a ketogenic diet for an individual to arrive at this state.

Such a large number of individuals remain captives to the conviction that glucose is the main wellspring of fuel. Therefore, they live in dread of coming up short on glucose. Yet, fat is the perfect vitality source and has been for the greater part of human advancement. That is the reason we have fat on our bodies! We really need just negligible glucose, most or all of which the liver can supply varying consistently. The pitiful actuality that starches and sugar are so modest and promptly accessible doesn't imply that we ought to rely upon them as an essential fuel source. It is this dazzle faithfulness to the "carb worldview" that has driven such huge numbers of individuals to experience the immense range of metabolic issues that take steps to overpower our human services framework.

Being a Sugar Burner

To comprehend being keto-adjusted, it is valuable to inspect being a sugar burner. A sugar burner can only with significant effort get to put away fat for vitality. That implies a sugar burner's muscles can't oxidize (or separate) fat. I know, the sprinter's magazine you are perusing says that your body consumes glucose for vitality, which is why long-distance runners have a colossal pasta supper the night prior to a race and afterward have oats for breakfast. I did that for a considerable length of time and ran some really great long-distance races, be that as it may, I was overweight and had a ton of joint agony.

I basically needed to be snared to a glucose IV trickle since I was constantly ravenous or "hangry" (hungry + furious). At the point when I went two, three, or four hours without nourishment, or even— might I venture to state it—avoided a feast, the individuals around me expected to keep an eye out! I was the meaning of an enduring sugar burner.

The human body developed to rely upon the oxidation of fat for most of its vitality needs. In a keto-adjusted body, fat tissue discharges a lot of unsaturated fats four to six hours in the wake of eating and during fasting, because the muscles can use them for fuel. But since I continued eating bananas, granola bars, and other carbs, my cells were consuming sugar, not fat. When my glucose was spent, yearning would set in once more, and I would go after one more banana.

On the off chance that you are a sugar burner, you can't process the fat you eat for vitality. The hindering symptom is that progressively fat—from carbs, recall, not dietary fat— is put away than consumed. Sadly, sugar burners wind up increasing a ton of body fat. A low proportion of fat-to-sugar oxidation is a strong indicator of future weight gain.

A sugar burner depends on a fleeting wellspring of fuel for vitality. You can store just around 50 to 90 grams of glycogen, the capacity type of glucose, in your liver for vitality transformation, which truly isn't a great deal. You can likewise store glycogen in your muscles, a procedure that shifts a considerable amount from individual to individual (competitors generally have bigger stockpiling destinations on the off chance that they train with starches). You can't store glycogen particularly, be that as it may, except if you include the grams of sugar in the tidbits in your pockets. For instance, an extremely fit man with a 12 percent muscle to fat ratio who weighs 160 pounds has more than 19 pounds of fat to consume for oxidation, yet the glycogen in his muscles and liver is restricted to around 500 grams. Would you Or maybe have 19 pounds (8,618 grams) of vitality or 500 grams of vitality? I pick the more extended enduring vitality source.

Another significant issue with the restricted extra space for glycogen in our bodies is that while you're sleeping, you can't eat to renew this glycogen. So when sugar burners rest, their bodies come up short on glucose and start separating protein — muscle and bone—to make more glucose. After some time, this causes less lean mass and adds to issues like osteoporosis.

The Keto Diet for Women

The Keto Diet, or Ketogenic Diet, can be attempted by the two people. This diet depends on a high admission of protein and fat, for example, meat, fish, olive oil, eggs, what's more, limited quantities of vegetables. Ladies can encounter various wellbeing benefits with this diet including hormonal parity, weight reduction and even an antiaging impact. You ought to counsel your primary care physician before embraced this diet as it tends to be healthfully prohibitive. A multivitamin and mineral ought to be taken to enhance the Ketogenic Diet.

Does the Keto Diet Work for Women?

The appropriate response is yes! In the years that Dr. Cabeca has been utilizing the keto diet to help treat ladies, particularly those in perimenopause or menopause, she's barely ever observed the diet fall flat to create benefits. Her customers and patients have encountered weight reduction, improved blood sugar control, better quality rest and decreased menopause manifestations like hot flashes or night sweats.

Dr. Cabeca thought of the idea of joining a soluble diet with a keto diet after gauging the benefits of low-carb eating on one hand, with a portion of the negative input she was accepting from customers on the other. Albeit huge numbers of her customers experienced weight reduction rapidly and dependably while decreasing their admission of carbs, some moreover detailed managing symptoms like queasiness, weariness, and blockage due to the keto diet. The keto diet includes finding a good pace percent of day by day calories from wellsprings of solid fat, a significant change for a large portion of her patients who were acclimated with running on carbs, caffeine and sugar for vitality. It turned out to be certain that something different must be balanced in request to forestall the symptoms related to the keto diet. This is the point at which she thought of the plan to concentrate on reestablishing alkalinity first and principal.

Normal Questions Regarding the Keto Diet for Women:

1. How precisely does a basic diet fit into a keto one? Also, for what reason is that so significant for ladies?

While a ketogenic diet standardizes (glucose) levels and can support you keep up or arrive at a sound weight, an antacid diet is beneficial for its enemy of maturing impacts— particularly bringing down inflammation, boosting detoxification, and advancing hormonal parity, resistance and the sky is the limit from there. Conventional ketogenic diets, as a rule, miss the significant factor of reestablishing alkalinity. For some patients, the key is to arrive at a soluble pH first before starting keto in request to forestall feeling fomented, on edge, awkward or excessively ravenous.

How does an antacid diet work?

A basic diet bolsters by and large wellbeing — including diminishing indications identified with barrenness, PMS or menopause — by assisting with adjusting your inside pH level and increment supplement assimilation. Eating nourishments that are high in key minerals yet not very acidic can diminish normal side effects or clutters by advancing an increasingly basic condition, the common and favored condition of the body. Research shows that keeping up an increasingly basic pee pH level can secure solid cells and improve gut wellbeing. Otherwise called "basic debris diets," diminishing causticity, (for example, from espresso/caffeine, liquor, reuned grains or prepared meats) has benefits for the cardiovascular framework because of how it forestalls plaque development in veins, can help decline kidney stones, serves to keep up bone mass and is beneucial for decreasing muscle squandering because of maturing.

What kind of negative wellbeing impacts may an excessively acidic pH level add to?

A couple include: bone misfortune, muscle misfortune, and higher defenselessness to visit contaminations or ailments. One approach to follow if your body is adjusting admirably to an antacid diet is trying your pee pH level. The pH scale ranges from 1–14, with seven being unbiased and anything higher than seven creatures soluble. The objective is to in a perfect world have a pee antacid pH level between of 7.0–7.5 (a number that is marginally more basic than acidic).

2. Will a soluble keto diet forestall the absence of vitality and opposite symptoms that a few feel when they attempt low carb dieting?

For the most part likely, yes. The task is concentrating on eating a basic diet, notwithstanding a low-carb keto diet will significantly assist control with siding impacts for some ladies (and men as well!). The explanation is a result of high supplement admission, upgraded detoxiúcation and decreased dependence on "uppers" like caffeine (some in any event, overdosing on caffeine) and sugar for vitality.

3. What different variables ought to be considered, other than somebody's diet, that can inûuence their pH level?

While it's a critical factor, your diet isn't the main variable that influences your pH level and hormones. Different elements that influence alkalinity, besides the nourishments you eat, include: the degree of stress you manage every day, how much rest you get daily, the measure of daylight introduction you get and the degree of natural danger you're presented to.

4. Intermittent fasting (IMF) is regularly suggested working together with a ketogenic diet. Yet many marvel whether IMF fits for ladies or safe.

As indicated by Dr. Cabeca, "Fasting is a key part of a sound diet and has numerous enemies of maturing impacts." specifically Dr. Cabeca prescribes fasting to ladies during or after menopause because of its enemy of maturing impacts. For instance, a recent report distributed in the Journal of the American Medical Association found that when ladies went 12.5 hours among supper and breakfast (a typical type of fasting), the medium-term quick appeared to help improve resistant framework working to the point that it decreased their hazard for bosom disease. For what reason is discontinuous fasting beneficial for ladies, particularly if they're in perimenopause or menopause? Fasting permits the body to take a break from stomach related capacities and rather to concentrate on fundamental fix work and to procure the numerous different benefits of rest. At the end of the day, when fasting, the body's vitality assets go towards therapeutic work (like fixing tissue what's more, adjusting hormones) as opposed to stomach related procedures like delivering stomach corrosive to separate nourishment.

She has discovered that when ladies stick to having a lighter supper and afterward avoid eating for around 13–15 hours among supper and breakfast, they experience upgrades in their weight, glucose control, and so on. She prescribes that ladies take a stab at abstaining from eating after 8 p.m. or then again try different things with eating just two suppers for each day, with tea or stock between dinners to help control hunger. Another choice is to have a go at skipping supper through and through on 1–2 days out of every week. For most ladies, while endeavoring IMF, it's not prescribed to nibble between suppers except if the lady is exceptionally dynamic, (for example, a competitor in preparing) or managing a hormonal issue such as adrenal burnout.

5. To what extent should a basic keto diet be followed?

It's ideal to move toward this adjustment in eating as an approach to feel much improved and become more advantageous, as opposed to as a "prevailing fashion diet" or weight reduction fast fix. Dr. Cabeca suggests giving it a half year to test the impacts, remembering that some experimentation is normal along the way. The diet ought to in a perfect world be drawn closer in step-wise design, concentrating on soluble first before including fasting and the keto viewpoint.

Ketogenic Diet

Could Eating Too Much Protein Affect Your Kidneys?

The Effects of a Carbohydrate Deficiency

Symptoms of Protein-Only Diet

The Ketogenic Diet includes eating fats and proteins while taking out basically all starches. The main allowed starches are vegetables, for example, verdant green plates of mixed greens, and generally speaking, your starch consumption must be kept beneath 50 g for every day. When your body is denied of starches, it goes into a state known as ketosis in which both dietary and overabundance muscle versus fat is changed over into ketones in the liver and used to fuel your mind and muscles. This diet powers your body to fuel itself through fat, not sugar and conveys with its various medical advantages for ladies. The high-fat ketogenic diet has numerous advantages. As per an examination distributed by the National Institute of Health, ladies put on a high-fat diet had more significant levels of estradiol, dehydroepiandrosterone and testosterone than ladies put on a low-fat diet. These hormones are indispensable for female wellbeing. Estradiol manages development hormone for tissue and regenerative organs, dehydroepiandrosterone is significant for regenerative wellbeing and memory and goes about as an upper and testosterone assists with reinforcing bones and muscles and improves sex drive.

The Ketogenic Diet is a strong fat misfortune diet for ladies. Jonathan Desprospo of bodybuilding.com says that the primary advantage of the Ketogenic diet is the capacity to cause your body to utilize fats for fuel, helping you to lose fat quickly. Due to the high protein admission, the Ketogenic Diet will have a muscle saving impact on your body says Desprospo. This implies bulk, which is basic for keeping the digestion working ideally, will be safeguarded. As indicated by an investigation distributed by the "Diary of

American Medical Association," ladies put on the Atkins Diet, which is a low starch, high fat and protein diet, lost more weight than those put on the Zone, Ornish or LEARN Diets.

Being in a condition of ketosis has different advantages for ladies. As per Michael Eades M.D., high protein diets have the impact of cleaning our cells. After some time, our cells become soaked with "garbage" protein matter. Eades states that a low-starch or then again ketogenic diet inverts this and fundamentally cleans the cells, causing an enemy of maturing impact on your body.

HIGH FAT OR NO FAT

This subject makes certain to come up when we are discussing the ketogenic diet. Fat has consistently been criticized as one of the primary drivers of cardiovascular infection. This was in no little part because of the Seven Countries Study done by Ancel Keys, where he validated research discoveries from seven extraordinary nations that at last made him connect utilization of fat with an expanded danger of cardiovascular diseases. It was a great instance of simply concentrating on inquire about numbers that bolstered his theory and dismissing the other divides which may have repudiated his hypothesis. This examination prompted an exacting overall clasp down on fat utilization and low-fat diets, on the off chance that you recollect those, turned into extremely popular. Fortunately, the current look into has, at any rate, exposed a portion of the connection among fats and heart issues. What most present-day researchers and nutritionists can concede to is that there are a few fats that are not unsafe to the body. Truth be told, fats are named as a basic macronutrient, accurately in light of the fact that our bodies need them to work. Let us presently investigate the fats which are regarded as useful to the human framework, since they will be significant parts of the ketogenic diet!

Monounsaturated fats, of which I will not exhaust you with the stuffy concoction definition, are normally present in fluid-structure at room temperature in their most perfect state however will in general set when you place them in crisp limits. You would be unable to discover any individual who gives a negative survey on this specific fat nowadays since it has been named a solid heart fat. A smidgen of incongruity is influencing everything here since it wasn't too quite a while in the past that all fats were named as one of the primary drivers of coronary illness, and at present, we have the monounsaturated sort liable for bringing down the dangers of heart issues!

The greater part of the monounsaturated fats that we expend come as avocados, just as olive oil. It is likewise present in almonds, cashew nuts, as well as eggs. Another wellspring of monounsaturated fat, which would likely become one of our instinctive decisions of nourishment, would be dim chocolate. Keep in mind; we are discussing chocolate where the cocoa content is at any rate 80% - the higher the better. Dim chocolate may take some becoming acclimated to, particularly for people with a sweet tooth who like milk chocolate. The distinction in the effect on wellbeing, in any case, makes everything advantageous to grasp the switch. Without the overabundance sugars present, and with a comparing increment in the valuable cocoa content, dull chocolate makes a difference with bringing down terrible LDL cholesterol just as improving the cardiovascular hazard profile of the customer. Other than the advantageous monounsaturated fats, dim chocolate additionally contains a rich degree of accommodating cell reinforcements that work to control ceaseless incendiary ailments just as improve psychological capacity.

Another fat which has gotten some positive logical writing would be the polyunsaturated assortment. Like its monounsaturated kin, it is typically found in fluid-structure at room temperature, while refrigeration would by and large set these fats. Polyunsaturated fats are considerably more vulnerable to oxidation from warmth and light, and this is the place the core of the issue lies.

Oils from soybean and corn, just as the sunflower, are rich wellsprings of omega-6 polyunsaturated unsaturated fats, and these fats should lower your LDL cholesterol. In any case, it is entirely expected to have both warmth and light in bountiful amounts when we look at most oil extraction strategies. The equivalent would likewise remain constant for fish oils, which are wealthy in omega-3, the different celebrated polyunsaturated unsaturated fat. Issues in handling, which involve excessively warmth and light, unavoidably oxidizes the past solid fats.

At the point when oxidized, the polyunsaturated fat turns into an entirely unexpected creature. Oxidized fats are known as trans fats or franken fats. They bring totally no medical advantages to the body yet significantly increment cardiovascular hazard frequency just as boosting cancer-causing development inside the body. Free radical levels are additionally raised when we expend trans fats. On the off chance that there was a substance on earth that I would not suggest, this would most likely top the list. To exacerbate the situation, trans fats happen in minute amounts normally, which implies we presumably wouldn't experience the ill effects of its belongings on the off chance that we left things to nature. Shockingly, the vast majority of the trans fats destroying their route into our body frameworks are of human build, by method for oil extraction what's more, handling. The greater part of the singed and handled nourishments accessible in the market are likewise subordinates of vegetable oil, because of its modest and prepared accessibility. We would do ourselves a major kindness in the event that we were to avoid these vegetable oils truly. Rather, there are sure oils and substances that are more reasonable for high warmth cooking and we will address those later. For the time being however, our most logical option for getting quality, unadulterated omega-6 and omega-3 polyunsaturated unsaturated fats would most likely be through eating natural pine nuts and pistachios. Greasy fish like trout and salmon would be extraordinary wellsprings of omega-3, taken crude in the Japanese sashimi style or softly barbecued in Mediterranean flavors would likewise be acceptable. For the people who are contemplating getting omega-3 enhancements like fish oil, it would be best on the off chance that you could go for makers who use forms which include as meager warmth and light as could be expected under the circumstances. In such circumstances, in some cases going old fashioned and conventional may be superior to any brand new techniques.

The key is to pay special mind to the nonattendance of warmth, and light, just as weight, in the extraction strategy for the fish oil. Nonattendance of synthetic added substances is additionally a major in addition to in guaranteeing you get natural, non-debased fish oil. It might appear to be a difficult task, and I would need to state it is from no modest quantity of investigating on my part that I found this specific brand of fish oil which happened to be removed in the customary Viking way, barring current obstacles like light, warmth, weight and compound added substances. Simply type "Rosita fish oil" into any web crawler and you ought to have the option to find a good pace organization's site.

I might want to state here this is the thing that I use by and by, and I have seen great outcomes from supported utilization of their additional virgin cod liver oil. I am in no way, shape or form associated to the organization nor am I embracing it. This is simply something I might want to impart to any individual who is searching for quality fish oil supplements in an offer to help their omega-3 admission. Omega-3 unsaturated fats are significant for cerebrum wellbeing, and studies have indicated that patients who endured horrendous mind wounds saw improved recuperation when eicosapentaenoic corrosive (EPA) and docosahexaenoic corrosive (DHA), two of the more conspicuous omega-3 acids, were legitimately presented through the intravenous framework. Omega-3 acids are additionally significant in managing the body's incendiary reaction.

Their essence produces calming substances which goes a long path in offsetting the hurtful impacts of sugar and trans fats present in the current diet. Omega-6 acids are fundamental for appropriate incendiary capacity too, since they contain triggers which set off the aggravation response in the body. An appropriate incendiary reaction is required in the body to go about as a sort of firewall or guard against outside pathogens and destructive substances that may somehow or another hurt us. The key here is the harmony between omega-3 and -6 acids, where the ideal proportion is viewed as two sections omega-3 to one section omega-6. You need to have the option to revitalize your body's barrier powers when adversaries show up at the entryways, yet in a similar setting, you additionally need to be capable to stand them down after the infections are squashed. Having the body's guard keyed up for a really long time is an ideal formula for ceaseless aggravation.

The last sort of fat that we are taking a gander at would be immersed fat. This is where the more genuine discussions and contentions would occur relating to the effect that this fat has on human wellbeing. Some staunch devotees of the hypothesis that interfaces immersed fat to coronary illness despite everything hold out that cutting down on immersed fat would significantly help lower cholesterol just as the dangers of cardiovascular infection. Others, in any case, point to expanding proof that soaked fat makes little difference to the advancement of heart infection. Immersed fat gets its terrible notoriety for heart issues because of the reality that it is thought to stop up conduits through the development of atherosclerotic plaque. The plaque contains fat and cholesterol, just as other substances, and it makes for an entirely feasible case to express that fat is fundamentally answerable for the arrangement of this perilous plaque. But that things aren't generally what they appear.

In the event that we dive somewhat more profoundly into the capacity of atherosclerotic plaque, the simple hypothesis of immersed fats stopping up veins, similar to squander sticking up the kitchen sink and channels, may appear to be a play feeble. Consider it: whenever immersed fats were actually that awful, people in the period of our grandparents and extraordinary grandparents would have been subjects of a coronary illness pestilence! They were expending red meat, grease, cheeses and other full cream dairy items that were all high in immersed fat. How can it be that our progenitors discovered it okay to have these full-fat nourishments with no significant therapeutic issues? However, we would be reconsidering things while devouring similar nourishments? The issue, it appears, lies not with fats, yet with our cutting edge fixation on sugar. Sugar has been legitimately recognized as one of the primary driver of ceaseless aggravation and the essential offender for a lot of weakening afflictions that appear to prosper in the created world. Diabetes, Alzheimer's, also, even metabolic disorders have all been ascribed in entire or to some degree to the raised nearness of sugar in our cutting edge diet. As it occurs, aggravation likewise happens in our organs and supply routes, and our bodies, being this astounding biochemical supercomputer, will at that point convey mending substances to those aggravated zones in an offer to redress or cordon off the issue. This is what occurs on account of our courses, experiencing and harmed the sugar assault, the plaque that structures is made by our bodies to conceal the regions in trouble and attempt to recuperate them. Picture a cut or a cut on your arm, as it is mending, a scab would shape to shield the injury from re-opening, which is actually what's going on with the arrangement of blood vessel plaque. The plaque shapes in an offer to permit the body to mend the influenced supply routes. More regularly than not however, the body would, in any case, be exposed to high measures of sugar through diet and recuperating is certainly debilitated. At the point when the zone is rendered hopeless, the body at that point endeavors to shield this harmed segment away from the remainder of the solid framework, and that is when atherosclerosis starts decisively.

A few people may at present, marvel about the degrees of cholesterol and fat found in the blood vessel plaque and point to that as a wellspring of concern. It may come as nothing unexpected to realize that cholesterol is one of the more significant fixings required when the body has a need to mend itself. This is the reason cholesterol is recorded as a fundamental substance for the human body. There are numerous who are worried about elevated cholesterol readings, however low cholesterol levels are too a reason for restorative concern since it suggests a potential issue in the body's mending capacity.

Soaked fat likewise assumes its job in guaranteeing appropriate nerve motioning just as improving the invulnerable framework's presentation. This invulnerable framework guideline becomes critical when we are discussing mending forms in our body. With the nearness of cholesterol and soaked fat in blood vessel plaque clarified, I would deduce this should set most minds calm about immersed fat! Keep in mind, a wide range of fat are required by the body for fundamental capacity, so it would truly be counterproductive for a diet to embrace low fat. Keep in mind, the cerebrum is made of generally immersed fats, furthermore, immersed fats are required for it to keep up ideal capacity. The myelin sheath, a protecting substance for legitimate nerve transmissions and flagging, considers cholesterol and fat its increasingly significant developmental parts.

Immersed fat nourishments would be a wellspring of adequate stock for these structure squares. At this crossroads, we realize that fat is required and is, truth be told, an essential fixing in huge numbers of the significant body forms required to continue life.

Additionally, we could most likely help ourselves out and oust the connection between sound, natural fats and cardiovascular sickness. Note that I said sound and natural fats. Trans fats or franken fats despite everything ought to stay on the highest point of your watch list for restricted substances! So feel free to appreciate the solid fullfat nourishments you find galore in the ketogenic diet with a genuine feeling of serenity, in light of the fact that this is an extraordinary opportunity to recover the body into an ideal metabolic state and transform it into a characteristic fat consuming machine for sure!

BENEFITS OF KETO DIET FOR WOMEN

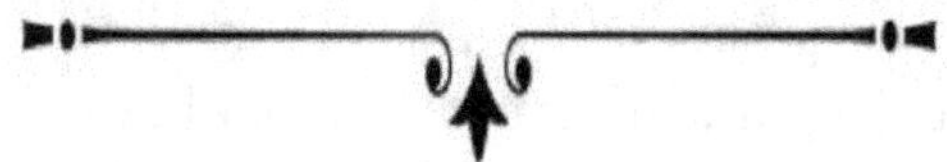

1: The Keto Diet Eliminates Glucose Highs and Lows t the point when you expend sugars, your body needs more insulin so as to process those carbs. The body's reaction to sugary carbs isn't simply in light of sugary treats. Regular nourishments like bananas, apples, bread, and even the basic sweet potato additionally require expanded insulin creation. After some time, particularly if your diet contains elevated levels of starches, you may turn into insulin safe, which makes it harder to deal with your glucose. On keto, on the other hand, you'll have progressively adjusted glucose levels — and thus, you'll encounter various key advantages that make this diet completely fantastic.

It will bring down irritation all through your body.

This is something that causes a speedy weight drop when you initially go into ketosis, however weight reduction isn't the just advantage! With lower levels of aggravation, you'll have less agony, less stomach related problems, and by and large feel superior to anything you did only a couple of brief days prior.

You won't pine for nourishment the manner in which you used to.

Glucose highs and lows can leave you wanting your preferred sweet treat at the very least potential minutes. Fortunately, at the point when you're in ketosis, those desires decline. Rather, your longings will normally become increasingly moderate. Accordingly, your body a greater amount of what it truly needs so as to remain more beneficial.

You won't gorge like you used to.

Let's face it: when we've attempted to diet, we've all fizzled intensely by going on a gorge session at any rate once at the day's end. Rather than getting the outcomes you were seeking after, you finished up feeling enlarged, awkward, and disillusioned in yourself — yet it's definitely not your issue! These gorge assaults are commonly the aftereffect of fluctuating glucose.

You'll have the option to get more fit easily.

At the point when you aren't managing extraordinary desires and battling through glucose highs and lows, your body is in prime position for you to shed pounds. Not just that, you'll rapidly find that you try not to need to give it as much exertion as you did on past diets. You won't be hungry constantly, and you'll have the option to appreciate numerous nourishments that you beforehand thought were untouchable when you were attempting to diet. It's a success right around!

2: The Keto Diet Balances Hormones for Better Sex and Fertility

Did you realize that not eating enough fat can cause fruitlessness in ladies? Cholesterol makes the entirety of your hormones. Eating the correct nourishments will guarantee that you're ready to deliver the correct hormones to help keep you more advantageous — and that doesn't simply reestablish your fruitfulness. It can likewise prompt better sex. Eating unfortunate fats prompts expanded PMS issues and worries during menopause. By eating well fats like the ones you find a workable pace the keto diet, then again, you'll find a workable pace period with fewer indications.

Subsequently, you'll be more joyful and feel more advantageous in any event during your period. In case you're experiencing menopause, you'll see that adhering to a keto diet can help decrease menopause side effects, from hot flashes to crabbiness. Your hormones will be progressively adjusted. You'll have better sex, appreciate expanded vitality and drive, and find that you're in a superior situation to appreciate time with your accomplice. You'll diminish issues with your period. Do you have PCOS? Amenorrhea? From sporadic periods to periods that are missing inside and out, the keto diet can help tackle a large number of the issues you manage each month, diminishing side effects furthermore, assisting with adjusting your richness. As examined in a past article, following the keto diet can make it simpler for you to get pregnant, remain pregnant, and produce the perfect measure of milk while you're breastfeeding — all of which make it definitely justified even despite the exertion.

3: The Keto Diet Helps Optimize Mind Function

Nobody enjoys that fluffy, foggy feeling like you're battling just to think. At the point when you select the keto diet, you'll find that mind mist is a relic of days gone by, and you're ready to work at more beneficial, progressively ideal levels. Consider: The mind is made of cholesterol and fat. That implies that the cerebrum needs sound fats to work at top proficiency — and without them, you may rapidly start to see the negative impacts.

Fat admission helps diminish or forestall side effects of wretchedness. Despondency can, in reality, be a typical symptom for ladies who are on a low-fat diet, while a diet high in sound fats can cause you to feel more joyful, more advantageous, and better arranged to manage everything on your plate for the afternoon. The expansion in great cholesterol implies an expanded generation of the hormones that control your temperament, leaving you more joyful.

You'll have the option to think quicker. With a diet high in sound fats, you'll have the option to think and react quickly and handle whatever difficulties are tossed in your direction for the day. That disappointing cerebrum haze will vanish, leaving you feeling much better prepared regardless of what you're managing. Stunningly better, you'll be in the perfect situation to stay aware of everybody around you — and even, in numerous cases, beat them.

4: The Keto Diet Offers Expanded Nutrients for Better Overall Wellbeing

Do you wind up becoming ill constantly — regularly for what you feel is alongside no explanation by any means? Is your insusceptible framework bizarre? In case you're sick of conveying around a crate of tissues or running from individuals who give even the scarcest indications of ailment, the keto diet can help improve your insusceptible framework and make you more advantageous. There are numerous advantages of the keto diet that can help improve your wellbeing, including:

Numerous nutrients are fat dissolvable and assimilate better when you eat a high-fat diet. Without those indispensable fats, you can take nutrients all you need; however they won't essentially make it into your body, where they can offer you the advantages you need. On a high-fat diet, they ingest better, permitting you to encounter all of those significant advantages. Your gut finds a workable pace break. You won't eat to such an extent, so your body won't need to process to such an extent. Subsequently, your gut will find the opportunity to recuperate itself. This abatements side effects of swelling and intestinal uneasiness.

As you become more beneficial, you'll have the option to get thinner all the more effectively. Fat-consuming potential increments as your wellbeing improve, placing you in a superior situation to let the pounds slide directly off.

You'll have the option to go long periods without eating. High-fat diets imply that you'll feel full more, which diminishes the occasions you'll require to nibble for the day. You'll additionally find that going longer between suppers helps lower irritation.

5: Get in Better Touch with Your Body for Lifelong Wellness

At the point when you're ready to encounter the other four key advantages, you're ready to get in better touch with your body, generally speaking, which can help lead to deep-rooted health. Being in contact with your body matters! It offers you various basic advantages. You comprehend what does and doesn't work for you. At the point when you're associated with your body, you have a superior thought of what is working for you, pushing you to accomplish the outcomes you need and abatement pointless side effects. This permits you to build up a superior arrangement for diet, exercise, and by and large health. You get off the dieting thrill ride. Rather than getting in shape for a brief time of time, just to pivot and picking up it once more, you'll have the option to leave on another way of life that will assist you with meeting your long haul objectives.

You'll feel as if you're a piece of a similar group with your body. Rather than having a feeling that your body is the foe and you need to battle it to arrive at your objectives, you'll have the option to jump in agreement and work with your body in a manner that will assist you with accomplishing your wellness and health objectives. You'll feel things better and be in a superior by and large situation to appreciate life on your terms — without battling your body to do it!

As a lady, the keto diet is one of the best things you can accomplish for yourself. At the point when your body is in ketosis, you'll have the option to arrive at your objectives — not only for weight reduction, yet in huge numbers of incredible aspects. In case you're attempting to lose weight, battling with cerebrum mist, or need to quit feeling lousy constantly, consider how the keto diet can help transform yourself to improve things.

Advantages of the Ketogenic Diet for Women Over 50

"Eat more beneficial and get more exercise" is the go-to guide for pretty much any weight or wellbeing concern today. The inquiry is the thing that "eat more advantageous" signifies to every person. A great deal of that has to do with hormones, and maybe nobody realizes it superior to ladies beyond 50 years old. One way of life change, specifically, is to present what is known as the Keto Diet. It's not so much a diet; however a condition of the body, actuated by a protein-rich menu. What's more, it has some novel highlights that are accounted for to affect wellbeing just as weight positively.

Fundamentally the same as the Atkins diet, many have utilized it to get in shape and make other wellbeing upgrades basically by confining the measure of sugars in their diet. There's a ton of a buzz about it, so we should see if we can sparkle some light on what that buzz is about.

1: Fast Hassle-Free Weight Loss

As we age, our digestion commonly eases back down around age 50, making it harder to get in shape. One of the best advantages of the keto diet is that numerous individuals begin to get in shape immediately. By limiting the measure of carbs taken in, our bodies would then be able to utilize fat stores for fuel.

At first, a ton of water weight is lost; however the uplifting news is, after moving beyond the principal period of the diet our bodies change. Sugar desires die down, vitality levels rise and many even report more concentration and honed mental sharpness. There are no exacting point frameworks to follow or costly packs to purchase. If this arrangement sounds great to you, begin by loading up on explicit nourishments on your next basic food item run. Get things like:

Evade every single handled nourishment like bread, chips, and grain. Drink a lot of water to keep yourself hydrated for the duration of the day. To get more data, look at this rundown of ketoaccommodating nourishments and the fundamental principles of the ketogenic diet. Obviously, similarly as with any diet or exercise plan, consistently counsel with therapeutic High protein meat like chicken, steak and fish Breakfast nourishments, for example, frankfurter, bacon (indeed, bacon!!) and eggs Full-fat dairy, for example, substantial cream and curds

Unreasonable Advantage Over Men: Women Learn Hidden "Joy Button" New spinach greens and non-dull vegetables proficient before you start to settle on sure it's a savvy decision for you by and by.

2: Reportedly Helps Manage Type 2 Diabetes

For those determined to have diabetes or prediabetes in their 40s or 50s, the ketogenic diet may help control blood glucose levels pushing ahead. As a result of the diminished sugar consumption, it's simpler for a body to direct blood glucose levels. This permits them to maintain a strategic distance from sugar spikes and makes it simpler to create and manage insulin levels.

3: Combats Fatigue

Getting more established and having more slow digestion regularly prompts feeling tired all the more frequently. A decent method to battle exhaustion is to exercise and keep an abundance weight off. With a keto neighborly diet, you can nibble as much as you need (on the correct nourishments, obviously) without feeling hauled down in the wake of eating a feast. Being in a condition of ketosis, or fat-consuming mode explicitly targets obstinate tummy fat. Midsection fat prompts instinctive fat, which crushes inward organs and keeps them from working appropriately.

4: Improves Neurological Health

Maturing can put us at an expanded hazard for dementia and certain types of it, for example, Alzheimer's sickness. Concentrates show a potential connection between a keto diet and a deferral in the beginning of Alzheimer's. This could be since an over-burden of glucose in the circulation system can make concentrating troublesome, which can influence your memory. Keeping levels consistent and in the ordinary range improves intellectual capacity nearly right away.

Weight gain is regular for some ladies in their 50s and past. The ketogenic might be a useful instrument to improve wellbeing and shed pounds as well! On the off chance that the exports exceed the cons in your book, converse with your primary care physician and check whether the keto diet is directly for you.

HOW KETO BRINGS WEIGHT LOSS FOR WOMEN OVER 50

One of the principal things that we generally lose when we set out on the ketogenic diet is undoubtedly water weight. The body stores glucose as fat fats, yet, there is a little stock of glucose that is put away as glycogen, which comprises of general water. Glycogen is intended to supply brisk blasting vitality, the sort that we need when we are run or lifting loads. As we cut carbs, the body goes to glycogen as the primary pool of vitality supply, which is why water weight will be lost in the underlying stages. This underlying explosion of lost weight can be a spirit sponsor for some, and it is a decent omen for what is to seek people who adhere to the keto diet. On a side note, water weight is effectively lost and picked up. This implies for people who see a few outcomes on the keto diet at first and afterward choose to get off the fleeting trend for reasons unknown, the odds are their weight would swell back up once carbs turn into the day by day caloric backbone.

For the rest who stay with the ketogenic diet, what occurs next will be the muscle to fat ratio's consuming instrument, which is liable for the dumbfounding weight misfortune results seen by many. The fundamental reason is as yet the equivalent, in that fat fats are presently enacted as wellsprings of vitality by the body's organs and cells, prompting a characteristic condition of fat misfortune and henceforth going with weight decrease.

Fat consuming isn't the main motivation behind why weight reduction is seen on the keto diet. Craving concealment and improve satiety after dinners are additional reasons why people can get more fit better while on a diet. The aphorism of eating less what's more, moving more has consistently been one of the long-standing precepts in weight misfortune. The entire thought is to make a calorie shortfall with the end goal that the body is required to depend on its put away supplies of vitality to compensate for the required consumption. On paper, that sounds simple and straightforward, however for any individual who has experienced circumstances where you have needed to control your eating on a ravenous stomach intentionally, it could be as troublesome as scaling Mount Everest!

With the ketogenic diet, you realize that you will have regular craving concealment, because of the modification of the hormones which control sentiments of yearning and completion. Other than that, the nourishment that we regularly expend while on the diet likewise assists with the weight reduction. Fats and protein are known to be more satisfying and satisfying than sugary carbs. At the point when we change to a high fat diet while eliminating the carbs, we accomplish two things basically simultaneously. Moving back on carbs, particularly the sugary stuff, lessens the drive to eat because you feel like it, not because you are really hungry. Lifting the fat admission likewise makes the satiety impact a lot snappier what's more, lets you feel full. This is a piece of the motivation behind why numerous keto dieters state that they can go on over two or even two suppers per day without feeling the scarcest spot of craving.

On our keto feast plan, we represent a day by day caloric admission that reaches from 1,800 to 2,000 calories, so we don't generally use calorie limitation all together to decrease weight. Actually, when you are encountering totality and fulfillment from your dinners, those modest and guiltless looking tidbits that possess the time in the middle of dinners won't include much in your life! Think about it: doughnuts, chips, and cakes, which are the common go-to snacks, get cut out, basically on the grounds that you are more averse to surrender to indulgent yearning caused fundamentally by those equivalent sugary treats! That goes a truly long path in cutting overabundance calories, which would some way or another have been changed over to fat tissue.

To summarize it, the ketogenic diet considers dinners without the common calorie limitation of other weight reduction diets. It likewise gives some assistance in making hunger concealment impacts so you don't need to fight with those devious cravings for food! There is likewise the nonappearance of carb desires, which can possibly wreck any diet. This lets us appreciate regular weight reduction with as meager interruption to our day by day lives as would be prudent. No calorie counters should be conveyed, no requirement for an inconvenient six to eight dinners every day, and unquestionably no peculiar or amusing activity schedules required. At the point when you couple that with the satisfying keto high-fat suppers, you arrive at a circumstance where craving may find a workable pace become an outsider surely.

Finding a workable pace genuine appetite resembles likewise comes as another positive turn off. On a carb-rich diet, we get occurrences of appetite in light of the fact that our glucose levels will in general change uncontrollably as our cells become bit by bit insulin desensitized. Sugar additionally expands the inclination to eat on motivation, which can truly crash any diet! At the point when we cut down on carbs and increase on the fats, we would truly need to pay attention when we feel any appetite aches, because those future legitimate signs that your body needs refueling.

OTHER GOOD STUFF FROM THE KETOGENIC LIFESTYLE

Something other than having the capacity to turn around type 2 diabetes, the ketogenic diet has various valuable impacts which I have recorded beneath. This will be a great inspirational sponsor or update during examples along with the keto venture when troubles arise and quitting turns into a to some degree agreeable choice. Try not to surrender! These are the beneficial things anticipating you toward the finish of the rainbow!

Regular yearning concealment – Like what has been explained beforehand, this component of the keto diet comes in extremely convenient when you will probably accomplish some weight reduction. You would now be able to do as such without experiencing insane cravings for food.

Feasible weight reduction and support – Another thing that makes them go for the ketogenic diet is the way that you for all intents and purposes don't need to look out for any unexpected weight bounce back or insane weight gains on the off chance that you keep on track with the diet. The mechanics of ketosis doesn't permit that to occur, and of course, we are discussing ordinary dinners here, not seven or 8,000 calorie nourishment plans which would agitate the weight reduction process. You can still gain weight in the event that you eat excessively!

More clear contemplations in the psyche – Due to the neuroprotective advantages that ketones really present on the cerebrum, one of the extra favorable circumstances of going keto would encounter a more honed and more clear personality. Thought forms are contacted with greater lucidity, without the mind haze that is normal for people on prepared carb-rich diets. Ketones are consuming all the more effectively as fuel likewise adds to this upgraded mental clearness.

Experience better and progressively stable temperaments – When the body enters ketosis, the ketones created for vitality additionally help with the harmony between two synapses that administer the mind: GABA, otherwise called gamma-aminobutyric corrosive, just as glutamate. GABA serves to quiet the mind down, while glutamate goes about as an energizer for the cerebral framework. The stunt to a sound and cheerful mind is to keep these two substances in right parity, and ketones positively help to accomplish that end.

Improve vitality levels and explain incessant exhaustion – Instead of having roller napkin spikes in your vitality levels, the ketone energized body will permit you to experience expanded vitality levels that stay pretty much steady as long as you have your dinners when yearning hits. Ceaseless exhaustion additionally turns into a nonissue because of the raised degrees of vitality. Regardless of whether the incessant exhaustion is a side effect of different infections, many find that however, it doesn't leave totally, the tiredness improves on the keto diet.

Get your aggravation levels down – When you guarantee that you have the sufficient parity of omega-3 fats, these solid polyunsaturated fats help to decline the incendiary reaction in the body framework. This makes for good news to the individuals who are experiencing incessant provocative sicknesses. In addition, the carb limitation would most likely observe your sugar consumption coming route down, which will help in lessening aggravation too.

Lower your triglycerides perusing – With a decreased carb admission, the degree of triglycerides in the blood would consequently be brought down. Triglycerides structure at the point when we have abundant calories, for the most part from carbs, with the goal that the body can start the way toward putting away the unrequired vitality as fats. At the point when the body is powered transcendently by ketones and not by glucose, the requirement for creating triglycerides really diminishes because of the adjustment in dietary propensity. On keto, you eat when you are extremely ravenous, and not in light of uncontrollably fluctuating blood sugar levels just as the alarm call of carbs.

Improve your lipid board readouts – Going keto will, as a rule, see your HDL cholesterol going up while the LDL cholesterol levels will go the other bearing. There might be a few cases where you will see both HDL and LDL levels increment, bringing about a general increment in cholesterol levels.

A few people have communicated worry on this issue and I might want to expand somewhat more on this. LDL and all out cholesterol levels may turn into raised for some who go on the ketogenic diet, however this ought not completely crack you out! Consider it right now: your body has been harmed metabolically during that time of eating handled and sugary carbs, the increment in cholesterol is really a sign that the body is experiencing a mending cycle so as to standardize metabolic capacity. At the point when the harm is to a great extent fixed, LDL and absolute cholesterol levels will in general beginning tilting descending. Everybody's body is unique, thus also is the time taken for the fix to be affected. Some may get brings about months, while others may need a year or two to get the ideal levels.

Less oxidative pressure – The ketogenic diet is liable for expanding the cell reinforcements present in the body, while likewise straightforwardly diminishing the oxidation that is experienced by the body's mitochondria. With supported cancer prevention agent movement while on the keto diet, free radicals will, in general, make some harder memories in exacting oxidative harm on our bodies. Less oxidation, as a rule, implies that our cells and organs work better and appreciate a more drawn out period of usability. This moreover implies that there could be an opportunity to draw out our life span since oxidation, being one of the prime explanations for maturing, sees its action being limited somewhat while on the ketogenic diet.

These are just a portion of the advantages that you will find a workable pace you go keto. I would have wanted to place in more data, particularly where the ketogenic diet has effects affected ailments like malignancy, polycystic ovary disorder, non-alcoholic greasy liver ailment, and neurodegenerative infirmities like Parkinson's and Alzheimer's.

Be that as it may, the goal of this book has consistently been to give flavorful and flavorful culinary answers for the keto dieter. It may be a smart thought to pop over to my other book, Ketogenic Diet.

The Step by Step Guide for Fledglings: Optimal Path to Effective Weight Loss, where I go into additional subtleties on the different advantages of the keto diet. In it, I additionally give a simple to follow, bit by bit guide which would slip you into ketosis, just as featuring those quick and dirty bits of valuable data to watch out for. Certainly of incentive to the keto novice, and a helpful book to have around as an update for the more prepared keto dieter, you can get the duplicate here in the US and here in the UK.

The ketogenic diet is an amazing new device to hit the standard as of late. This style of eating has significant information behind it, indicating that it can support fat-consuming, decrease irritation, help subjective execution, and that's just the beginning. What has not

CHALLENGES WOMEN OVER 50 FACES DURING KETO DIET AND HOW TO VOID THEM

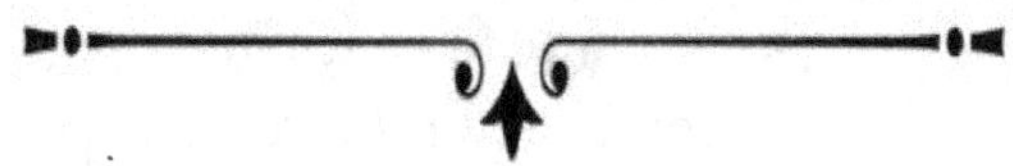

been secured very enough are basic keto symptoms and how you can stay away from them to make the best of this amazing eating style.

Even though there can be a wide range of symptoms that show while turning out to be keto-adjusted, they all come from comparable fundamental issues. Right now, diagram what those fundamental issues are, their related keto reactions, and basic methodologies to conquer them so you can become keto-adjusted as easily as could reasonably be expected.

Three Primary Causes

Although there is an assortment of indications that can emerge during keto adjustment, they for the most part show from a similar three basic causes. Hypoglycemia (low glucose), HypothalamicPituitary-Adrenal (HPA) hub brokenness, and electrolyte/mineral deficiencies.

While these three causes are unique, they are in reality, all related. While turning out to be keto-adjusted initially,your body has been running on sugar for a considerable length of time. At the point when you out of nowhere change to fats, your body needs to fabricate the phone apparatus important to produce and use ketone bodies as a fuel source. This implies as opposed to creating huge amounts of ketones from the earliest starting point, the vast majority experience hypoglycemia for a timeframe. With hypoglycemia comes a disturbance in cortisol flagging which is the thing that records for the HPA pivot brokenness. At long last, HPA hub brokenness prompts an expansion in the emission of minerals from the body in the pee.

Together these three causes can make a wide range of keto symptoms. When you get them, however, a tad of Hypoglycemia as I briefly referenced as of now, hypoglycemia is the first fundamental reason to add to reactions during keto-adaptation. This is because the body essentially doesn't have the foggiest idea of how to consume fat for vitality yet. During the adjustment stage, individuals ordinarily feel cerebrum mist, weariness, wooziness, extraordinary appetite, peevishness, and melancholy.

In spite of the fact that hypoglycemia is typically first and foremost, these keto reactions ought to die down inside long stretches of starting a

Keto Flu

Keto flu is one of the most notable keto reactions. Keto influenza is actually what it seems like, the beginning of influenza-like indications that emerges soon after starting a ketogenic diet. This incorporates indications like weariness, runny nose, sickness, and cerebral pain. Keto influenza is a great appearance of hypoglycemia that can be redressed with straightforward systems that I will diagram in the blink of an eye.

Numerous individuals find that during the starting phases of a ketogenic diet, they experience extraordinary nourishment desires. These nourishment longings are ordinarily for high-sugar food sources and will in general, truly challenge your resolution. This is an exemplary hypoglycemia reaction also. The mind specifically requires heaps of vitality for ordinary capacity. At the point when it gets a sign that you are hypoglycemic, a frenzy reaction happens on account of a hidden observation that you are starving to death (regardless of whether deliberately you know you're most certainly not). Now your mind starts to disclose to you that, "YOU NEED IMMEDIATE ENERGY NOW OR YOU'RE GOING TO DIE"!

This is the point at which you have extraordinary sugar desires. Fortunately, when you start to deliver ketones for vitality, this frenzy reaction quiets down. Basic difficulties that ladies more than 50 may confront/keto reactions. Also, with the correct dinner plan and enhancements, you can stay away from the greater part of these by and large. First, however, we should investigate what may occur. In the age of the "corpulence scourge," more research than any other time in recent memory is centered around deciding sheltered, powerful, and enduring approaches to help forestall or turn around undesirable weight gain.

Furthermore, considers have discovered that one potential arrangement is following an exceptionally low sugar diet called the ketogenic diet. The keto diet diminishes the body's stockpile of glucose—which is normally acquired from eating starch substantial nourishments like grains and sugar—rather compelling the body to utilize fat for vitality. That may sound like other low-carb diets, yet there is one key keto differentiation: Instead of attention on heaps of protein, the keto diet underscores solid fats, generally from ketoaffirmed nourishments like coconut or olive oil, spread, meat, avocado, and eggs.

Thus, the keto diet doesn't simply help with weight reduction. It's additionally been appeared to diminish the hazard for diabetes or coronary illness, secure against certain neurological clutters, and improve psychological capacity. Be that as it may, that doesn't imply that receiving the keto diet will be all going great, either. For some, the change from a high-carb diet to one that is worked around solid fats and a lot of vegetables can trigger some side impacts.

What Side-Effects Can We Expect From Ketosis for more than 50 ladies?

The keto diet is sheltered as long as you stick to explicit rules and ensure you don't keep your body from imperative supplements. While the symptoms recorded on this page are normal, they are connected to your body's digestion rolling out some extreme improvements.

In case you're thinking about receiving the keto diet to help improve your general wellbeing, be exhorted that you may run into at least one of the accompanying difficulties. The uplifting news, in any case, is that the majority of these will probably disseminate inside half a month—or even sooner if you follow my recommendation.

1. Clogging

Since you'll be eating far fewer starches than you're utilized to while on a keto diet, you'll likely additionally be diminishing the measure of fiber in your diet. This can add to different stomach related changes, including obstruction. To help keep things "moving," drink a lot of water and make a point to eat an assortment of low-carb plant nourishments all through the day, particularly highfiber veggies like verdant greens, cooked cruciferous veggies and avocado.

You may likewise need to enhance with a stomach related catalyst, especially one that contains the catalyst lipase. Lipase is the essential catalyst that separates dietary fats, which will help with the entirety of the additional avocado and coconut oil you'll likely be expending.

2. Low vitality

Numerous metabolic changes need to occur in your body with the goal for you to switch from utilizing fat for fuel rather than glucose. And keeping in mind that this procedure unfurls, it's normal to encounter times of exhaustion, shortcoming, and mind mist as your body saves vitality for the previously mentioned metabolic procedures.

One approach to help keep your vitality up is to ensure that you're not dried out and that you're likewise getting enough fundamental supplements, particularly electrolytes. Numerous keto dieters find that adding salt to their suppers and having some bone soup regularly assists with reestablishing a portion of the electrolytes that are lost during ketosis, counting magnesium, potassium, and sodium. Bone stock additionally supplies various other significant supplements and amino acids, while diminishing potential symptoms like muscle squandering, cerebral pains, squeezing, and fits.

What's more, you should expect to rest at any rate eight hours out of every night and go lighter on your calendar during this progress period, which ought to keep you from feeling even progressively pushed and run down. On the off chance that you can't rest soundly, attempt these common tips to fall sleeping quick, or have a go at taking around 400 milligrams of magnesium citrate before bed.

3. Muscle shortcoming

Notwithstanding feeling more worn out than ordinary on the keto diet, you may likewise understand diminished quality, trouble recouping from an intense exercise, as well as a general shortcoming. Therefore, I prescribe sparing any extraordinary instructional courses for when you're feeling more grounded and more empowered—particularly in case you're likewise managing indications of hypoglycemia (another potential symptom of ketosis), which can cause transitory insecurity, dizziness, and perspiring.

So how might you battle this potential shortcoming? First off, make certain to eat enough protein to fuel your body—however, not all that much. On the keto diet, the aggregate sum of protein required isn't high, about 1.3 grams of protein per kilogram of perfect body weight. On the off chance that you speculate you're not eating enough by and large, have a go at having more non-boring veggies and fat, rather than more protein, as an overabundance can prompt lack of hydration, state of mind swings and kidney issues (also terrible breath).

To recharge sodium levels—if hypoglycemia is an issue—you may likewise need to attempt having a glass of water with around one-quarter teaspoon of Himalayan or regular ocean salt blended in.

4. Expanded longings

As indicated by a 2007 report that showed up in the American Journal of Clinical Nutrition, "One significant favorable position of the ketogenic diet is that it permits the calorie admission to be cut definitely without delivering insatiable craving." So even though your general hunger might be diminished on the keto diet, actually your yearnings for carbs or sugar probably won't be. Nourishment inclinations and instilled dietary propensities can set aside some effort to change, so it's expected that you may manage some brief side effects of "withdrawal" as you expel certain solace nourishments from your diet. As a rule, this may be a greater amount of an intense subject matter than a physical indication, so show restraint toward yourself and recollect that your taste buds are fit for evolving. Make certain to eat enough calories as a rule, what's more, permit time for your inclinations to get themselves straightened out, which will occur as you begin feeling better generally speaking. Eating progressively solid fats, fiber, and sufficient measures of lean protein will help kick those longings, as will ordinary servings of probiotic-rich, aged nourishments.

5. Testiness

Numerous individuals don't understand exactly how associated their stomach related framework is to their apprehensive framework. At the point when your diet changes, so do the creation of hormones and synapses that influence how you feel, rest and act. You may see that for the primary couple a long time on the keto diet, you're feeling unmotivated and for the most part, horrendous, yet this doesn't imply that the diet is doing hurt.

To put it plainly, it takes effort for your mind to adjust to its new vitality source (recollect: fat, not carbs), so keep it together. If manifestations like the absence of rest, drowsiness, or waiting migraines are adding to your poor temperaments, have a go at getting more magnesium from nourishments like verdant greens, avocado, and salmon to help. You should intend to eat at any rate two cups of crude, green, verdant vegetables every day, notwithstanding other non-bland veggies that you appreciate.

Additionally, recall that contemplation, exercise, and journaling are extraordinary, non-nourishment approaches to improve your state of mind quickly.

Wooziness and Drowsiness

At the point when you are hypoglycemic while additionally not being completely keto-adjusted, you have a vitality deficiency inside the body. This is a transient adjustment that can prompt an assortment of keto symptoms. During this time, you will probably feel discombobulated and languid because of the general absence of vitality. You may feel particularly mixed up after remaining because of circulatory strain dysregulation and improper cortisol reaction (HPA hub dysregulation which we'll discuss without further ado).

Diminished Strength and Physical Performance

During keto-adjustment, your body is figuring out how to use a new fuel source that it has not needed to use previously. The muscles (alongside the mind) contain huge amounts of mitochondria for vitality generation that must currently figure out how to use ketones as a vitality source.

During this time, you will probably feel a significant drop in quality and capacity to apply physical vitality as one of the short term keto reactions. Fortunately, when you become adjusted, you should see extreme upgrades in these territories that are much more prominent than when you were sugar-adjusted!

Approaches to Overcome Keto Side Effects For Women Over 50

1. Eat More Alkaline Foods

How precisely would women be able to eat a diet that is both antacid and permits them to remain in ketosis? Are there any nourishments on the keto nourishment rundown to abstain from eating even though they are actually "low carb"?

Dr. Cabeca feels it's basic to include bounty low-carb alkalizing decisions (foods grown from the ground) to a ketogenic diet for ideal beneúts and anticipation of reactions. She particularly prescribes supplement thick nourishments like avocado and dull, verdant greens. Here is a rundown of no-carb to reasonably low-carb nourishments that ladies (and men, as well) can remember for a soluble keto diet: Greens like kale, chard, beet greens, dandelion, spinach, wheatgrass, horse feed grass, and so forth.

Other non-boring veggies or herbs like mushrooms, tomatoes, avocado, radishes, cucumber, jicama, broccoli, oregano, garlic, ginger, green beans, endive, cabbage, celery, zucchini and asparagus. In a perfect world attempt to expend a decent part of your produce crude or just softly cooked, (for example, steamed), as crude foods can help supply elevated levels of alkalizing minerals Include different superfoods like maca, spirulina, ocean veggies, bone stock and green powder blends that contain chlorophyll.

Solid keto neighborly fats like coconut oil, MCT oil or virgin olive oil. Fats found in wild caught fish, grass-sustained hamburger, confine free eggs, nuts, seeds and natural grass-encouraged margarine are likewise great increments to your diet. Littler measures of dull plants like sweet potato, turnips and beets can likewise be included in the diet, even though these ought to ordinarily be kept to bring down sums due to containing more sugar and carbs.

In the event that conceivable, attempt to devour antacid water. Basic water has a pH of 9 to 11, making it a preferred alternative over faucet water or puriúed filtered water that progressively acidic.

To diminish your admission of poisons and synthetic concoctions, it's ideal to buy natural produce at whatever point conceivable and to pay extra for grass-nourished, unfenced creature items. Plants that are developed in natural, mineral-thick soil will, in general, be additionally alkalizing and supply the most value for-your-money.

While they may be alright from time to time, by and large, it's not prescribed to eat a lot of organic products or high-carb veggies that taste extremely sweet to look after ketosis. While working towards arriving at a progressively antacid, ketogenic state (ketosis), attempt to limit or avoid these nourishments:

All wellsprings of included sugar Grains (even entire grains)

Most dairy items (now and then modest quantities of full-fat yogurt/keúr or cheddar can be alright)

Attempt to have eggs, lentils and nuts like peanuts in modest quantities, since these are more acidic than different proteins. Maintain a strategic distance from prepared meats including cold cuts, or industrial facility ranch-raised meats, which advance sharpness.

Caffeine Liquor Other prepared nourishments that contain loads of sodium, sugar, manufactured fixings and Úllers (see our when there's no other option keto inexpensive food list)

2. Attempt "Crescendo Fasting" (or different kinds of carb cycling)

There are different approaches to rehearse irregular fasting on keto, including some that are less liable to trigger symptoms like weakness or desires. Crescendo fasting offers you a reprieve from fasting consistently, yet is still useful for accomplishing the beneúts of IMF. Dr. Cabeca and different specialists, for example, Amy Shah, M.D., encourage their patients to check their urinary ketone levels (utilizing ketone strips) and to target testing decidedly for ketones around three days out of each week.

Work towards cycling fasting days so you're fasting on 2–3 nonconsecutive days out of each week (for example, Tuesday, Thursday and Saturday). Stick to just light exercise or yoga on fasting days to lessen feeling depleted or hungry, keeping higher power exercises for your non-fasting days. This methodology takes into account progressively dietary and way of life "balance" because the objective isn't to eat 100 percent "impeccably" constantly.

3. Oversee Stress and Rest Enough

Tending to the significant wellsprings of physical and enthusiastic worry in your life is fundamental for recuperating fundamental hormonal lopsided characteristics and fruitfulness issues. Expect to get 7–9 hours of rest every night to reset your hormones day by day. Absence of rest can truly influence your absorption, hunger and vitality levels!

A few different ways to oversee pressure include: getting enough moderate development and exercise, yoga as well as reflection, going for moderate strolls outside, journaling or perusing, being progressively social by joining some gathering or group, resting more, petition, and so on.

4. Forestall Constipation with More Fiber and Water

In the event that your body is making some hard memories changing in accordance with a keto diet, attempt to eat more fiber from veggies, nuts or seeds and drink enough water to help hydrate the digestive organs to ease obstruction. Dr. Cabeca prescribes beginning the day with a major glass of high temp water with lemon and a spot of cayenne pepper.

Through the rest of the day, attempt to drink a large portion of your weight in ounces of water day by day (for the model, 65 ounces or somewhat more than 8 glasses on the off chance that you weigh around 130 pounds). Taking probiotics is additionally a smart thought because of how this recharges the gut with sound "great microorganisms."

Precautionary measures Regarding the Keto Diet for Women

Beside obstruction and introductory longings for carbs or sugar, opposite reactions you may experience while progressing to an antacid keto diet (particularly in case you're likewise starting fasting) can incorporate "keto flu" indications like period issues, adrenal or thyroid issues, weakness or low vitality levels.

While here and there, it may feel like things are deteriorating before they show signs of improvement; these side effects should resolve inside half a month too long periods of following the tips and program referenced previously. This is particularly valid in the event that you attempt to stay dynamic (walk, in a perfect world outside, for at least 20–30 minutes every day), rest soundly and decline pressure. Drink a lot of water, homegrown tea or bone soup to forestall lack of hydration, and back off of activity in case you're feeling under-filled.

It's additionally worth referencing that on the off chance that you have a background marked by unpredictable periods, any sort of eating clutter, or a thyroid issue than it might be ideal to start this sort of dietary program as it were while being guided by your primary care physician or a nutritionist. Pregnant ladies or the individuals who are breastfeeding ought not to begin the keto diet to be protected. An expert can assist you with slipping into a basic keto diet in a moderate, safe way in case you're uncertain of how to do this on your way, giving you criticism so the diet won't adversely meddle with typical hormone generation, craving, rest or mental core interest.

Hypoglycemia Mitigation Strategies

As should be obvious, a significant extent of keto reactions are credited to hypoglycemia. These are my top techniques for tending to these issues.

1. Eat Every 3-4 Hrs: Eat every 3-4 hours when in the first place phases of a ketogenic diet. This will help keep you satisfied and glucose adjusted.

2. Drink Mineral Rich Drinks: Instead of plain water, drink mineral-rich refreshments between suppers. This incorporates natural soups or a top-notch electrolyte drink (like this one)

3. Hydrating and Mineral Rich Foods: Consume a lot of hydrating, mineral-rich nourishments and utilize salt liberally. I like to nibble on celery, cucumbers, and particularly ocean growth as these Sea Snax. These resemble ocean growth chips that taste incredible and contains many beneficial minerals.

4. Utilize Exogenous Ketones: Exogenous ketones are a phenomenal method to prepare the body to utilize ketones for fuel before our body is acceptable at making ketones. They likewise cushion hypoglycemic reactions by giving ketones the body can use for vitality as opposed to having a significant stress reaction when glucose drops. An extraordinary exogenous ketone item that additionally has adaptogens and electrolytes is Keto Edge

5. Use Magnesium Supplementation: If you follow these techniques and keep on feeling a significant number of these manifestations, consider adding a magnesium supplement to your routine. I would suggest taking the L-threonate structure, (for example, our Brain Calm Magnesium) in a 1 gram portion – 3x every day between suppers.

HPA Axis Dysfunction

The HPA Axis is a progression of three organs (Hypothalamus, Pituitary, and Adrenals) that are fundamentally answerable for managing our pressure reaction in the body. At the point when we experience hypoglycemia, as I referenced previously, the cerebrum goes into a crisis reaction to starvation. In expansion to sugar longings, the adrenals will discharge cortisol. Cortisol flags the arrival of putting away glucose in the body (glycogen stores) to give quick vitality. Given this reaction, glycogen amasses rapidly caught fire, hypoglycemia reoccurs, and the cycle proceeds. This is the place HPA pivot dysregulation advances the beginning of related manifestations while additionally intensifying hypoglycemia-related Sleep Problems With HPA pivot brokenness, you are probably going to encounter an interruption in rest. This is because cortisol is opposing to melatonin (which means it contradicts its capacity). At the point when the HPA pivot is distracted, cortisol levels start to fluctuate and meddle with the arrival of melatonin that happens at the evening.

To audit briefly, hypoglycemia animates the arrival of cortisol. Cortisol flags the arrival of put away glucose in the body, called glycogen, from the liver and muscle tissue. Cortisol is an invigorating hormone that can disturb rest if this reaction occurs around the evening time. These outcomes in either a sleeping disorder or extremely low-quality rest.

Despite the fact that this cortisol reaction is useful in crises, you need to attempt to limit it however much as could reasonably be expected during keto-adjustment and particularly around evening time.

Heart Palpitations

Numerous individuals will see heart palpitations during the early periods of keto adjustment. This can be ascribed to Hypoglycemia, HPA pivot brokenness, and mineral lopsided characteristics. During HPA pivot dysregulation, cortisol can turn out to be anomalous high. On the off chance that it stays high, the body will create cortisol opposition. To repay the body starts to emit higher measures of adrenaline which would then be able to cause sporadic heart rhythms.

Moreover, the loss of minerals that we are going to talk about can prompt a decrease in blood volume and weight that can make the heart siphon quicker or even unpredictably.

Supporting The HPA Axis

Like I said as of now, during the underlying adjustment period of a ketogenic diet, there is potential for the HPA hub to become dysregulated. During this time, it is worthwhile to play it safe to help the HPA hub as best as you can. These are my top techniques for HPA hub support during keto-adjustment to lessen keto reactions:

1. Glucose Balancing Strategies: Follow the glucose guideline techniques plot above. Hypoglycemia is one of the essential triggers of cortisol dysregulation so address this first!

2. Magnesium Supplementation: This is laid out above yet I need to address it again here. Magnesium is an incredible help for the HPA pivot. Magnesium L-threonate specifically is the main structure demonstrated to have the option to cross the blood-cerebrum boundary which implies it can apply its impact on the nerve center and pituitary organs.

3. Use Adaptogenic Herbs: Although this technique isn't completely essential, utilizing adaptogenic herbs can massively benefit the HPA hub and help assemble your versatility to push. By supporting the HPA hub and assisting with controlling cortisol levels, adaptogens may demonstrate extremely accommodating in moderating HPA pivot related symptoms.

Electrolyte/Mineral Deficiencies

Electrolytes and minerals serve the essential capacity of managing hydration while supporting legitimate nerve conductivity. During keto-adjustment, an overabundance of minerals are discharged through the pee due to HPA hub dysregulation.

This is because, notwithstanding cortisol, the HPA pivot is likewise liable for managing hydration levels through the maintenance and discharge of minerals. As it were, HPA pivot dysregulation can likewise prompt hydration dysregulation.

Moreover, there are basic keto reactions that happen that show from these lopsided characteristics.

Visit Urination

The most evident sign that your electrolyte/mineral equalization is being influenced is an expansion in pee. On a low-carb diet, insulin levels drop, which advances the discharge of sodium in the pee. Sodium maneuvers more water into the urinary framework which at that point is discharged too. This is an extremely ordinary one of the keto symptoms and a positive sign you are moving towards keto adjustment.

Also, as your body consumes glycogen stores in the liver and muscles, abundance water is discharged into the urinary framework. While disposing of this additional water is useful in discharging poisons from the body, you need to ensure you are taking in extra fluids, electrolytes, and minerals to dodge other related symptoms.

Blockage

The blockage is a key sign that you are not looking after electrolyte/mineral equalization during keto adjustment. The consistency of somebody's stool, and in this manner the capacity to pass that stool, is intensely influenced by its water content. Your general hydration levels similarly influence the water substance of your stool. Additionally, clogging may likewise be a reaction of an adjustment in your microbiome. Your gut microscopic organisms cosmetics is to a great extent controlled by the sorts of nourishments you eat. When making such an extreme change in your diet, your microbiome will change which can likewise briefly change your stools.

Likewise Consider: Certain nourishments can in general be increasingly helpful for the stoppage. Nourishments like eggs, cheddar, and nuts might be adding to clogging. Decrease admission of these in any event during the underlying periods of keto adjustment and check whether that has any effect.

Muscle Cramps

A typical one of the keto reactions individuals involved with the early stage is muscle cramps. On the off chance that you experience visit muscle cramps while turning out to be keto-adjusted this is likely because of irregular mineral characteristics.

As I referenced previously, minerals are vital for appropriate nerve drive conductivity. A muscle cramp is basically a misconducted motivation expedited by poor hydration and mineral equalization.

Keto Side Effects

Keeping up Proper Hydration and Mineral Balance

Presently you know about the physiological changes that add to visit pee, obstruction, looseness of the bowels, muscle spasms, and heart palpitations. Luckily, the procedures to alleviate these symptoms are very basic. With a little proactivity and arranging, these keto symptoms will probably be less of an issue. My top techniques for appropriate hydration and mineral parity are:

1. Super Hydration: Drink a lot of water, mineral-rich soups, and hydrating refreshments. You need to guarantee any poisons being discharged are flushed out adequately.

2. Utilize High-Quality Salt: Use a top-notch salt in liberal sums in the entirety of your dinners, This will include back in sodium, and other follow minerals that are discharged all the

more quickly during keto-adjustment. I like either Himalayan pink or a Celtic (dark) ocean salt as they are the most elevated in follow minerals.

3. Expend Mineral Rich Foods: Increase your admission of mineral-rich nourishments like verdant greens, celery, cucumber, and ocean growth. As I referenced previously, I love to nibble on Sea Snax as they give a lot of minerals and are ketogenic well disposed of.

4. Utilize a Magnesium Supplement: Unless you are encountering the runs, a magnesium supplement can work incredible for helping balance electrolytes and hydration levels. As should be obvious, magnesium can help ketoadjustment in numerous ways. Utilizing 1 gram of the Lthreonate structure 3x day by day is my general proposal. In the event that loose bowels happens, lower to on more than one occasion per day until it dies down.

KETO MEALS

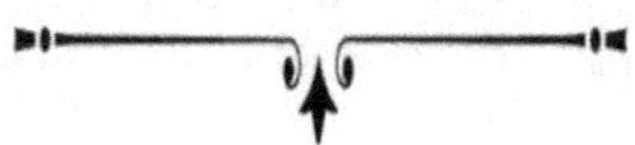

Presently we are finding a good pace of things! This part is going to begin by fleshing out the nourishments which you will get personally familiar with. Gracious truly, the greasy meats just as dairy items will highlight, and remember your greens and natural products! There will be another area on what sort of nourishments to cut down on so as to confine your carb utilization. The rundowns are intended to go about as a kind of simple groundwork with regards to keto inviting nourishments, so it gets simpler for you to select and recognize which nourishments are a great idea to go during feast times.

As we probably are aware, the standard ketogenic diet

macronutrient necessities are as follows

- 75% of Fats
- 20% Protein
- 5% Carbohydrates

At the point when we interpret this to an every day admission of 2,000 calories, that implies we are taking a gander at 1,500 calories from fats, 400 calories from protein and the staying 100 calories from carbs. With every gram of protein and carb yielding 4 calories, and every gram of fat yielding 9 calories, the entirety breakdown above will wind up with a day by day terrific figure of around 166 grams of fat, 100 grams of protein and 25 grams of carbs. These macronutrient numbers ought to be at the bleeding edge of your mind when you first start off with the ketogenic diet. Simply recollect, consistently attempt to hit your fat necessity, limit your carb admission, and consider the measure of protein you are getting into your framework.

On the off chance that your experience is in any way similar to mine, you will find that eating adequate fat is by all accounts an issue, at any rate in the underlying stages. This is somewhat because a parcel of the fat that you take in is available in fluid structures. Consider olive and coconut oils, or the spread and grease when warmed on the skillet, these are all high-fat fundamentals in the keto diet however they can be barely noticeable in light of the fact that they will never be the mains in a dinner. I found that keeping the rely on my every day fat numbers helped in expanding my fat admission. When you locate the fat check being somewhat low, 99% dim chocolate just as impenetrable espresso can push those numbers up nearer to where they should be. Obviously, there are numerous other high fat nourishments which can do the stunt also, so how about we investigate them!

Nourishments to Enjoy On The Ketogenic Diet

There are various kinds of nourishment that fall into this rundown. These nourishment thoughts unquestionably push for highfat substance, while simultaneously pressing other supplements and solid nutrients in for the body's utilization.

Meats And Animal Products – Focus on grass-sustained or field raised greasy cuts of meat and wild-got fish, maintaining a strategic distance from cultivated creature meats and prepared meats however much as could reasonably be expected. What's more, remember about organ meats!

- Beef
- Chicken
- Eggs
- Goat
- Lamb
- Pork
- Rabbit
- Turkey
- Venison
- Shellfish
- Salmon
- Mackerel
- Tuna
- Halibut
- Cod
- Gelatin
- Organ meats

Solid Fats – The best fats to expend on the ketogenic diet are monounsaturated and polyunsaturated fats, however there are a lot of solid immersed fats too. At the danger of seeming like a messed up recorder, stay away from trans fats. Perhaps "evade" isn't a proper word. Flee may be better. Flee from trans fats like you would the plague. That's all anyone needs to know.

- Butter
- Chicken fat
- Coconut oil
- Duck fat
- Ghee
- Lard
- Tallow
- MCT oil
- Avocado oil
- Macadamia oil
- Extra virgin olive oil
- Coconut margarine
- Coconut milk
- Palm shortening

Vegetables – Fresh vegetables are wealthy in supplements and low in calories, which makes them a superb expansion to any diet. With the ketogenic diet, notwithstanding, you should be cautious about carbs, so stick to verdant greens and low glycemic veggies instead of root vegetables and other bland veggies. I set avocados right now a few of us may remember it as a vegetable even though it really is an organic product.

- Artichokes
- Asparagus
- Avocado
- Bell peppers
- Broccoli
- Cabbage
- Cauliflower
- Cucumber
- Celery

- Kohlrabi
- Lettuce
- Okra or women's fingers
- Radishes
- Seaweed
- Spinach
- Tomatoes
- Watercress ☐ Zucchini

Dairy Products – If you can endure dairy, you can incorporate full-fat, unpasteurized, and crude dairy items in your diet. Remember that a few brands will contain a great deal of sugar which could build the carb content, so focus on nourishment names and moderate your utilization of these items. In the event that conceivable, go for the full-fat forms as these will have a less likely possibility of sugar being utilized to supplant the fat.

- Kefir
- Cottage cheddar
- Cream cheddar
- cheddar
- Brie cheddar
- Mozzarella cheddar
- Swiss cheddar
- Sour cream
- Full-fat yogurt ☐ Heavy cream

Herbs And Spices – Fresh herbs and dried flavors are a great method to season your nourishments without including any noteworthy number of calories or sugars

- Basil

- Black pepper
- Cayenne
- Cardamom
- Chili powder
- Cilantro
- Cinnamon
- Cumin
- Curry powder
- Garam masala
- Ginger
- Garlic
- Nutmeg
- Oregano
- Onion
- Paprika
- Parsley
- Rosemary
- Sea salt
- Sage
- Thyme
- Turmeric
- White pepper

Refreshments – You ought to dodge every single improved beverage on the ketogenic diet, be that as it may, there are sure refreshments which you can at present have so as to include a little more assortment to your selection of fluids other than old fashioned water.

- Almond milk unsweetened
- Bone stock

- Cashew milk unsweetened
- Coconut milk
- Club pop
- Coffee
- Herbal tea
- Mineral water
- Seltzer water
- Tea

Nourishments On The Moderation List

These nourishment things are incorporated here because they will, in general, have a higher carb check, so control is significant. Be that as it may, they are packed with other supplements and some of them additionally toss in that additional piece of fat to help toward your everyday fat admission!

Natural products – Fresh organic products are a fantastic wellspring of nourishment. Shockingly, they are additionally stacked with sugar, which implies they are high in starches. There are a couple of low-to direct carb organic products that you can appreciate in littler amounts; however you need to watch the sum you eat! Once in a while, it is truly simple to continue popping them into our mouths. "Nature's treats" is certainly a precise moniker for them. We can even now get their advantages and keep up ketosis with the perfect measures of utilization. A large portion of the nitty-gritty of the organic product the following is alright for you to have a cup or thereabouts, maybe a solitary cut or two on a routine, particularly when you are first beginning and are hoping to keep your carb tally low. As you advance and show signs of improvement handle of your carb edge, it is okay to build the amount of these nourishments while remaining inside your assigned carb limit.

- Apricot
- Blackberries

- Blueberries
- Cantaloupe
- Cherries
- Cranberries
- Grapefruit
- Honeydew
- Kiwi
- Lemon
- Lime
- Peaches
- Raspberries
- Strawberries

Nuts And Seeds – While nuts and seeds do contain starches, they are likewise wealthy in solid fats. The accompanying nuts and seeds are low to direct in carb content, so you can appreciate them as long as you watch your segment sizes.

Typically an ounce or a bunch of nuts would be a decent check to perceive how much you can eat and still remain in ketosis day by day.

- Almonds
- Cashews
- Chia seeds
- Hazelnuts
- Macadamia nuts
- Pecans
- Pine nuts
- Pistachios
- Psyllium
- Pumpkin seeds
- Sesame seeds

- Sunflower seeds
- Walnuts
- Nut spread

Nourishments To Avoid

With regards to nourishment, you ought to keep away from on the ketogenic diet, and there are hardly any significant classes to refer to.

Most importantly, you ought to maintain a strategic distance from grains also, grain-based fixings however much as could be expected since they are the most noteworthy in starches. Pick solid fats over hydrogenated oils and attempt to restrict your admission of bland vegetables and high-glycemic organic products. With regards to sugars, refined sugars like white sugar and dark-colored sugar are totally limited, and you ought to likewise maintain a strategic distance from fake sugars. Normal sugars like nectar, unadulterated maple syrup, and agave are not terrible for you, yet they are high in sugars. The best sugars to use on the ketogenic diet are powdered erythritol, stevia, and priest organic product sugar.

Stevia is a herb that is otherwise called the sugar leaf. This sugar comes in a few structures, and you have to ensure that whatever kind you purchase doesn't likewise contain a counterfeit sugar. Fluid stevia separate is normally the best choice; however you can likewise discover powdered stevia extricate. Another choice is powdered erythritol, which is removed from corn, and it is, as a rule, the best choice to use in plans for prepared products. As far as sauces and fixings, you have to peruse the nourishment name to see whether the thing is keto-friendly or not because brands contrast extraordinarily. As a rule, essential fixings like yellow mustard, mayonnaise, horseradish, hot sauce, Worcestershire sauce, vinegar, and oils are keto-accommodating. With regards to things like ketchup, BBQ sauce, and serving of mixed greens dressings, you should be careful of the sugar content present in them.

Here is a snappy rundown of a portion of the significant nourishments you'll have to stay away from on the ketogenic diet.

- All-reason flour
- Baking blend
- Wheat flour
- Pastry flour
- Cake flour
- Cereal
- Pasta
- Rice
- Corn
- Baked products
- Corn syrup

- Snack bars
- Quinoa
- Buckwheat
- Barley
- Couscous
- Oats
- Muesli
- Margarine ☐ Canola oil
- Hydrogenated oils
- Bananas
- Mangos
- Pineapple
- Potatoes
- Sweet potatoes
- Candy
- Milk chocolate
- Ice cream
- Sports drinks
- Juice mixed drink
- Soda
- Beer
- Milk
- Low-fat dairy
- White sugar
- Brown sugar
- Maple syrup
- Honey
- Agave

WHAT TO LOOK OUT FOR IN SOME KETO FOODS

Since this is especially filling in as a formula book, I figured it would be fitting to share a few hints and thoughts on what to pay special mind to when we are picking the more typical and mainstream keto nourishments for preparing our suppers.

Salmon – This greasy fish has constantly positioned high for me with regards to keto well-disposed nourishments. You may realize that it will generally be pressed with helpful omega-3 polyunsaturated fats, which lift cerebrum wellbeing and help with diminishing aggravation, yet it likewise has heaps of different supplements that the body needs.

Potassium and selenium are found in abundant sums with regards to salmon. Potassium is necessary to appropriate guidelines of circulatory strain too as the body's water maintenance. Selenium assists with looking after great bone wellbeing just as guaranteeing an ideal safe framework. Over this, salmon likewise contains solid degrees of B nutrients. These nutrients are vital for proficient nourishment to vitality preparing, just as keeping up the best possible capacity of both the body's DNA and sensory system. To finish it off, salmon has astaxanthin, a cell reinforcement that gives salmon tissue its ruddy pink tint.

This ground-breaking cell reinforcement assists with heart and cerebrum wellbeing, and may likewise be useful for the skin. To get a decent quality arrangement, the primary thing you should observe is the smell. New salmon, or any fish so far as that is concerned, won't generally have a scent. You can likely smell a tinge of the sea, yet crisp fish will not smell fishy. At the point when it is fishy, you realize that fish isn't for you.

Next up, focus on the eyes. Search for those with clear and sparkling eyes. Think about a famous actor who has teared up - those are the sort of eyes that best show what you are searching for. Never go for depressed or dry-looking eyes. Overcast looking ones are additionally a no-go with regards to crisp fish choice.

Balances and gills are additional territories which we need to focus on. Crisp fish have balances that look wet and entire, not torn and worn out. Their gills are brilliant red and clean, not earthy red and vile. Ultimately, on the off chance that you are permitted to, have a go at squeezing the fragile living creature and checking whether it skips back like how your own does. The substance which is discouraged and remains discouraged ought not to wind up in your kitchen.

For filet cuts, all the better you can do is focus on the shading just as how the piece looks. The shading ought to be energetic and brilliant. Fluctuated tones running from red to coral to pink are worthy, yet consistently recall that the principal thing is the brilliance of the substance. Next is to detect any breaks or breaks in the tissue itself. These are signs that the filet has been kept for some time and is no longer as new. Additionally, any pooling of water ought to likewise trigger alerts, since it implies that the substance structure has begun to separate, and the time has come to proceed onward to another piece.

Pork midsection – This is another plausible staple in the keto diet. I've discussed it in my other book; however, here I need to focus on helping you pick a great cut for preparing your dinners. Every 100 grams of pork tummy contains around 50 grams of fat. Pressing another 9 grams of protein and positively no carbs, you can be certain this is a decent nourishment thing to help your everyday fat check. Besides, it very well may be totally simple to get ready heavenly dinners with it.

While picking pork stomach, you should take a gander at the shade of the cut. Go for the slices that are ruddy pink to darkish red. Meat which is lighter in shading, for the most part, implies the freshness may have blurred. Turning gray or staining will unquestionably imply that rot has just set in and the meat ought not begotten.

The other thing you need to search for is the streaky white segments of fat present in the pork tummy. By and large, the more streaks it has, the better the marbling will be and that is uplifting news for you. Continuously guarantee that the marbling is white, because any yellow or grayish shading would speak to the meat that has likely passed its sell-by date.

Avocado oil – I should be straightforward here and state that this oil, for me, has been a later stage expansion when contrasted with olive and coconut oil. Additional virgin olive oil, just as the adaptable coconut oil have their legitimate places in the pantheon of staple keto nourishments, yet avocado oil may be giving them a run for their cash.

Avocado oil one, comprises of for the most part monounsaturated fat. This specific eccentricity attaches into a significant point. The oil is considered unquestionably increasingly steady than any of its polyunsaturated fat cousins, similar to vegetable oil and even extra virgin olive oil. Other than that, avocado oil is known to have a higher smoke point, something like 500 degrees Fahrenheit, than most vegetable oils. This makes it a significant expansion to the kitchen because the oil has higher protection from degeneration by heat. Extra the way that it packs a solid punch as far as nutrients, minerals, phytochemicals, and cancer prevention agents, you will understand this is one oil you can use for various applications.

A few people use it for hair and healthy skin, where the nutrient E rich oil is known to be effectively consumed without extra synthetic concoctions or other conceivably hurtful added substances. Including the oil into servings of mixed greens, vegetables, or natural products is additionally an incredible approach to support monounsaturated fat admission with almost no burden. You may even need to take a stab at drinking it crudely, however, it doesn't work for me as I saw it as excessively crude. Blending it up with some lime or garlic has continuously been what I like. Presently how about we talk a little on the most proficient method to approach picking the avocado oil. First up, we need to take a gander at the source or inception of the oil, which ordinarily implies we need to know where and how the avocados were developed. Right now, we need to search for a confirmed natural mark to realize that the avocados were developed with no manufactured added substances. This guarantees the oil got from the avocados don't contain any substances that could be hindering to your wellbeing.

Next, we have to take a gander at how the oil is extricated. Mechanical and concoction extraction strategies utilized for the most part include expanded warmth just as strong synthetic concoctions to compel out the oil from the squashed avocado mash. The drawback of this is the warmth and synthetic compounds may lessen the helpful supplements and nutrients present in the oil. To address this, chilly squeezing, which is known as the least dangerous technique out there, guarantees that the shading, smell, and taste areas near the first organic product as could be expected under the circumstances. You show signs of improvement of quality oil, and an expansion to that, appreciate more supplements.

The last thing we have to take a gander at is how the oil is refined or not. Truly, for best outcomes, cold squeezed oil that is grungy and gotten from affirmed natural avocados, would rank among the top levels, if not the top. The drawback is that the timeframe of realistic usability is short, and the oil smells… avocado-ish. That shouldn't be an issue on the off chance that you use it regularly, and you should, considering the medical advantages and comfort that it brings. The following best thing would be to have the oil normally refined, where the producers regularly do stress and sifting to expand the period of usability. Continuously recall, the more the oil is refined, the less sustenance it will give.

Before it slips my mind, I consistently choose oils in dull hued glass containers or tins. This is somewhat like additional virgin olive oil where the oil can go malodorous in the nearness of warmth and light. For avocado oil, however, most of the fats present comprise of the monounsaturated assortment, there still is a minor level of polyunsaturated fats. Consequently, better to decide in favor of alert what's more, go for dim shaded glass bottles.

Ghee – This substance has been around since the Ayurvedic times, and it has continuously been recorded as the cooking mechanism of decision. Ghee is explained spread, which means margarine that has been warmed and is liberated from lactose just as other milk solids. This likewise brings about a higher smoke point contrasted with margarine. It can go as high as 480 degrees Fahrenheit, which implies you can extremely profound fry or then again cook without the danger of oxidation which discharges hurtful free radicals.

Expulsion of the lactose is incredible news for the individuals who are lactose narrow-minded, yet still wish to participate in the nutty and rich flavor that accompanies spread. Ghee can be an incredible other option, and the taste may even be progressively tasty. Pressed with numerous fat solvent nutrients, it additionally contains short-chain unsaturated fats that support cardiovascular wellbeing just as help battle aggravation. Ghee likewise has the particularly favorable position of having the option to last around three to about a month at room temperature while it can keep for as long as a half year when refrigerated.

Ghee can be found in most supermarkets. Check for it in the oil area, albeit a few spots may have it in the dairy parcel. As with spread, you can generally attempt to go for grass-sustained assortments first to improve the supplement allow and diminish the opportunity of having potential added substances or synthetic compounds blended in. For me, I, for the most part, go for ghee stuffed either in tins or glass containers.

Fat – Lard is fat from pigs. Once criticized together with the various soaked fat nourishment sources, fat is appreciating a welllegitimized rebound! Every 100 grams of fat gives you around 30 grams of soaked fat, with polyunsaturated fat making up 10 grams and the monounsaturated assortment yielding around 40 grams. No, there is no mix-up. You understand it accurately. Fat really has more monounsaturated fat than immersed fat content. Little marvel why people from the previous ages truly depended on grease and for all intents and purposes utilized it for most stuff including cooking and heating.

Since we present-day society are coming round to fat by and by, it has been seen as one of the more extravagant wellsprings of nutrient D nourishments. You don't have to get all your nutrient D from the sun or fish, grease is likewise a scrumptious other option! On top of that, grease is additionally useful for high warmth cooking as a result of its higher smoke point which remains around 375 degrees Fahrenheit. There is additionally less possibility of rancidity or free extreme creation because of the nearness of immersed fat substance which gives grease that additional layer of fat soundness. Did I as of now notice that grease tastes incredible too? That is a point worth rehashing since there is only something about creature fat that gives nourishment an extremely rich furthermore, tasty surface.

Lamentably, fat being sold in markets and most stores aren't generally great since they have most likely experienced some type of hydrogenation in request to delay the timeframe of realistic usability. Delaying market fat's time span of usability comes at the cost of our own on the off chance that we decide to include it into our dinners. You truly ought to be hoping to get great fat from your butcher or meat merchant. Great fat, otherwise called leaf fat, is gotten from instinctive fat around the kidneys and midsection region of the pig. In the event that that has run out, you can go for the following best other option, which is grease that is marginally progressively strong and is gotten from between the back skin and muscle. Untreated or foul grease should consistently be refrigerated to keep up its freshness.

Ringer peppers – These brilliant vegetables not just include shading and a crunchy nibble to our day by day suppers, yet they likewise pack a serious sound punch in the supplements office. Plentiful in nutrients An and C, just as furnishing us with folate and nutrient K for included great measure, chime peppers help with boosting our invulnerable framework and keeping up tissue wellbeing. The cancer prevention agent lycopene, a sort of carotenoid that gives the peppers it's shading, is likewise dependable in assisting with lessening aggravation, just as being a functioning scrounger for the body's free radicals. It is likewise incredibly flexible, being superbly reasonable to serve crude or softly barbecued. All the more uplifting news? The carb mean 100 grams of ringer peppers remain at a measly 5 grams, of which 2 grams comprise of dietary fiber. We'll contact more regarding this matter of dietary fiber and how it impacts the carb tally, yet until further notice, simply realize that chime peppers have a strong low carb mean all the nutritious goodness it packs.

The secret to picking a ringer pepper that you would need to have on your supper table is simple - truly. Go for the ones with splendid, striking hues. The ones with lighter hues may show they aren't that ready yet. Any with wounds and staining ought to be saved and supplanted with those which have a polished sheen. Tenderly press the vegetable to feel for the snugness of the skin. One more thing to note is that a ready ringer pepper will really feel heavier than it looks. This is because it has not experienced dampness misfortune related to over readiness. Ringer peppers can be put away in the cooler for as long as 10 days, so make certain to pop them into the chill box once you bring them once again from your basic food item run.

The rundown above is intended to give some assistance with regards to the physical choice of these nourishments referenced. I am almost certain you might want to keep quality and new nourishments around in your kitchen and I trust this area would have gone some separation in helping you do that on a predictable premise. Next up, we will cover the 28-day supper plan that has been slyly arranged for you. Beginning with simple plans to let anybody get acclimated to the keto way of life, it advances in assortment throughout the weeks with the goal that you don't get exhausted with having similar suppers again and again. Allow's progression to up and investigate what we have for you!

KETO RECIPES

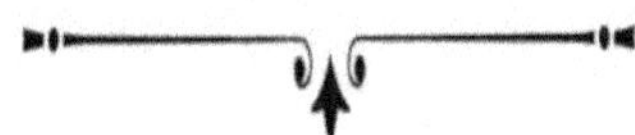

We needed to make it as basic as workable for you to get in the kitchen and stir up something uncommon, so you will discover every formula spread out in a simple to follow the design. Every start with a short introduction to the dish, trailed by the serving size and rundown of fixings. Keep in mind, this diet is intended to revive your adoration for nourishment not stifle it with rules and guidelines, so don't be hesitant to explore.

Utilize the fixings as general rules and adhere to the guidelines as best you can. You may not get everything impeccable first time, without fail yet that is the thing that makes it yours! Keep at it for an entire 30 days of eating and you will no uncertainty build up a couple of firm tops picks that you can transform into your claim to fame dishes after some time. Every formula closes with a breakdown of key dietary data, including a number of calories and a measure of fats, starches and protein.

Once more, this isn't to be fixated on. Nourishment is something to be delighted in, so on the off chance that you are going to keep a note of your admission levels than simply make it a general gauge.

Why no pics? This cookbook is brimming with fun and enhance, and doesn't take itself as well truly. The nourishment is entering your mouth, not a displaying challenge, and we don't like to energize unfortunate fixation on the introduction. So cook, explore, and appreciate. When you begin adoring what you are eating times will become something to anticipate. Accept this as support, go forward and cook to your heart's content!

KETO CREAM CHEESE PANCAKES

Truly, you can have flapjacks on the keto diet! You're one formula in and most likely previously starting to comprehend why it's so mainstream.

SERVES 8-10

Ingredients:

☐ 4 eggs, 4 oz. cream cheddar, relaxed 1 tbsp. sugar substitute, 2 tsp. vanilla concentrate 4 tbsp. coconut flour 1½ tsp. heating powder Almond milk varying

Directions

1. Consolidate the eggs, cream cheddar, sugar substitute, and vanilla with a blender or on the other hand blender.

2. Include the coconut flour and preparing powder. Join well. On the off chance that the hitter thickens following a couple of moments, add a little almond milk to thin it.

3. Warmth the electric frying pan to 325°F. Pour the hitter in 5inch circles.

4. Trust that the surface will air pocket, and afterward flip. Cook for 2-4 minutes longer, or until cooked.

5. Present with your preferred garnishes, or use for sandwiches.

Nourishing Info per Serving Calories: 100

- Fat: 8g
- Net Carbs: 3.5g
- Protein: 5g

SCRUMPTIOUS COCONUT FLOUR WAFFLES

Too ravenous and in a surge? This formula takes just couple of moments! Acknowledge the challenge to eat only one. It functions admirably with any fixing, and even the children will love it!

SERVES 5

INGREDIENTS

4 tbsp. Coconut flour, 5 eggs, isolated by white and yolk, 1 tsp. heating powder, 4-5 tbsp. granulated stevia or your own sugar, 3 tbsp. entire milk, 1 tsp. vanilla 4½ oz. margarine, liquefied.

Directions

1. Whisk the egg whites in a bowl until they structure firm pinnacles.
2. In another bowl, blend the egg yolk in with the coconut flour, the stevia or sugar, and the heating powder.
3. Include the softened margarine. Do so gradually, blending until the hitter is smooth.
4. Include the milk and the vanilla.
5. Join the blend of the principal bowl with the subsequent one, collapsing it in to keep the cushion of the hitter.
6. At the point when the waffle creator is heated up, pour in some waffle blend. At the point when it is brilliant dark colored, it's done.

Rehash until all the player is utilized.

NUTRITIONAL INFO PER SERVING

- Calories: 277
- Fat: 22g
- Net Carbs: 4.3g

- Protein: 8g

SOLID VEGETABLE BREAKFAST HASH

Bacon and veggies will make certain to light up your morning! Supplant the eggs with avocado for a sans egg elective.

SERVES 1

INGREDIENTS

- 1 medium zucchini
- ¼ cup white onion
- 2 oz. bacon
- 1 tbsp. coconut oil
- New parsley, cleaved 1 enormous egg
- Salt to taste

Directions

1. Cut the bacon, and strip and shakers the onion and zucchini.
2. Sauté the onion over medium warmth and include the bacon. Mix and cook until somewhat carmelized.
3. Add the zucchini to the dish, and cook for 10-15 minutes.
4. At the point when done, place the hash on a plate and include the hacked parsley.
5. Top with a seared egg or, for a sans egg adaptation, avocado.

NUTRITIONAL INFO PER SERVING

- Calories: 427
- Fat: 35g
- Net Carbs: 7g
- Protein: 17g

YUMMY AVOCADO AND SALMON BREAKFAST BOATS

Salmon and avocado are both acceptable and sound fat hotspots for your keto diet. Here, they join for a choice breakfast alternative.

SERVES 1

INGREDIENTS

- 1 avocado
- 1 oz. crisp goat cheddar
- 2 oz. smoked salmon
- 2 tbsp. lemon juice
- 2 tbsp. of natural additional virgin olive oil
- A scramble of ocean salt

Directions

1. Cut the avocado down the middle, evacuating the stone.
2. Blend the remainder of the fixings – the salmon, goat cheddar, oil, lemon juice, and salt - in a nourishment processor until they have a rich consistency, and spot the blend inside the avocado.

NOURISHING INFO PER SERVING

- Calories: 520
- Fat: 45g
- Net Carbs: 5g
- Protein: 20g

SAUSAGE CASSEROLE WITH VEGETABLES

The entire family will appreciate this magnificent breakfast meal. It takes not exactly an hour to make and keeps you fulfilled throughout the morning, so maybe one for a languid Sunday.

SERVES: 6

INGREDIENTS

2 cups zucchini, diced, ¼ cup onion, diced, 1 lb. pork frankfurter, 20 cups cabbage, destroyed 3 eggs, 2 tbsp. mustard, ½ cup mayonnaise, 1½ cups cheddar, destroyed 1 tbsp. dried ground sage Cayenne pepper.

Instruction

1. Preheat the stove to 375°F. Oil a goulash dish and put it in a safe spot.
2. In a huge skillet on medium warmth, cook the frankfurter and the veggies until delicate.
3. Spot the blend into the meal dish.
4. In a different bowl, blend the eggs, mustard, mayonnaise, sage, and pepper until consolidated well.
5. Add the ground cheddar to the egg blend and mix for 1 moment.
6. Pour the blend over the hotdog and vegetables in the goulash dish, and top with the cheddar.
7. Prepare the goulash for 30 minutes, or expel it when it is rising around the edges and the cheddar on the top is dissolved.

Dietary Info Per Serving

- Calories: 480
- Fat: 42gNet Carbs: 5g
- Protein: 20g

KETO LEMON MUFFINS WITH POPPY SEEDS

There's nothing superior to anything the flavor of lemon and poppy seed biscuits to revive you toward the beginning of the day. Quick to make and simple to store, they can be a piece of your breakfast (or late morning snacks) consistently. Furthermore, they're low-carb!

SERVES: 12

Ingredients

- ¾ cup almond flour
- ⅓ cup Erythritol
- ¼ cup Flaxseed supper
- 1 tbsp. preparing powder
- 2 tbsp. poppy seeds
- ¼ cup Butter, liquefied
- 3 eggs
- ¼ cup Heavy cream
- 3 tbsp. lemon juice
- Lemon get-up-and-go of 2 lemons
- 1 tbsp. vanilla
- 20 drops fluid sugar

Directions

1. Preheat the stove to 345°F.
2. In the interim, blend in a bowl the flaxseed feast, almond flour, erythritol and poppy seeds.
3. Include liquefied margarine, and blend in the eggs and overwhelming cream until it arrives at a smooth consistency.

Include the remainder of the fixings and blend.

4. Spot the hitter into the biscuit skillet (separated into 12) and prepare them for 18-20 minutes.

5. Expel from the stove and cool for around 10 minutes.

NUTRITIONAL INFO PER SERVING

- Calories: 130
- Fat: 11.5g
- Net Carbs: 1.7g
- Protein: 4g

BREAKFAST TACOS

A get and-go breakfast! You will be charmed by the crunchy cheddar taco shell what's more, the immense assortment of fillings you can use with it.

SERVES: 3

INGREDIENTS

- 1 cup mozzarella cheddar
- destroyed 6 eggs
- 2 tbsp. spread
- 3 portions of bacon
- 1 oz. cheddar, destroyed
- ½ an avocado
- Salt and pepper

COOKING INSTRCTIONS

1. Cook the bacon on a preparing sheet secured with aluminum foil at 375°F, until firm (12-15 minutes).
2. In the interim, utilize 33% of the mozzarella to cover the base of a nonstick skillet. Warmth for 2-3 minutes on medium warmth, or until the edges start to darker.
3. With a couple of tongs, expel the mozzarella from the skillet (it will presently be a taco shell). Rehash with the rest of the cheddar.
4. Scramble the eggs in the margarine. Mix every now and again, and add pepper and salt to taste.
5. Fill the shells with the eggs, avocado and bacon.

Nutrients Info Per Serving

- Calories: 440

- Fat: 36g
- Net Carbs: 4g
- Protein: 26g

CHEDDAR AND BACON OMELETS WITH CHIVES

Chives consistently give a remarkable flavor to your nourishment – and it's far better with cheddar and bacon! This formula is very simple and too delectable.

SERVES 1

INGREDIENTS

- 2 cuts of bacon
- 2 tbsp. bacon oil 2 eggs
- 2 stalks of chives
- 1 oz. cheddar Salt and pepper

Directions

1. Spot the bacon fat in a pre-warmed skillet on a medium-low warmth, and let it soften. Include the eggs, chives, salt and pepper. Mix softly.
2. Include the bacon once the edges are set. Cook for 20-30 seconds more.
3. Add cheddar to the omelet and overlap into equal parts. Flip over and warm through on the opposite side.

Nutrients Info Per Serving

- Calories: 460
- Fat: 40g
- Net Carbs: 2g
- Protein: 25g

PUMPKIN BREAD

In case you're a pumpkin darling and missing all the Halloween pumpkin treats, you're going to adore this portion. Each serving demonstrations like a tasty little protein bar.

SERVES: 10

Ingredients

- 1½ cups almond flour
- 3 egg whites
- ¼ cup granulated sugar
- ½ cup coconut milk
- ¼ cup psyllium husk powder
- 1½ tsp. pumpkin pie flavor
- 2 tsp. heating powder
- ½ tsp. salt **Directions**

- In a bowl, filter all the dry fixings. Spot a compartment with 1 cup of water into a preheated stove (350°F).
- Include the pumpkin and coconut milk to the dry fixings, and blend.
- Whisk the egg whites, and include them into the batter, collapsing cautiously.
- Spot the batter into a lubed portion skillet, and cook the bread for 75 minutes.

Nourishing Info Per Serving

- Calories: 120
- Fat: 9g
- Net Carbs: 3g
- Protein: 5g

SALTED CARAMEL CEREAL WITH PORK RINDS

This crunchy, salty-sweet blend will take your breath away toward the beginning of the day, which is badly arranged on the off chance that you've just barely put them on. In any case.

SERVES 1

INGREDIENTS

- 1 oz. pork skins
- 2 tbsp. margarine
- 1 cup vanilla coconut milk
- 2 tbsp. Substantial cream
- ¼ tbsp. ground cinnamon
- 1 tbsp. erythritol

Directions

1. In a container on a medium warmth, include the margarine and mix until caramelized.
2. Evacuate and include substantial cream and erythritol. Blend well and come back to the heat. Keep warming, blending continually until the ideal caramel shading is accomplished.
3. Include the pork skins and blend them in, being mindful so as to cover uniformly.
4. Spot them into a holder and put in the ice chest for 20-45 minutes to cool them down.

Nourishing Info Per Serving

- Calories: 510
- Fat: 50g

- Net Carbs: 2.7g
- Protein: 15g

RED CHOCOLATE DOUGHNUTS

Chocolate, vanilla and coconut meet up to make red velvet-like you've never tasted – and such that you won't feel unreasonably remorseful for eating one… or on the other hand two. SERVES 9

INGREDIENTS

For the doughnut:

- ¼ cup Erythritol
- ½ cup coconut flour
- 2 tbsp. cocoa powder
- ¼ cup coconut oil
- ½ cup coconut milk
- ½ tbsp. vanilla concentrate
- ¼ tsp. salt
- ¼ tsp. preparing pop
- 4 eggs
- ¼ tsp. apple juice vinegar
- ¼ tsp. fluid stevia
- 1 tsp. red nourishment shading **For the icing:**

- ¼ cup powdered erythritol
- 4 oz. cream cheddar
- 4 tbsp. spread
- 2 tbsp. overwhelming cream
- ½ tsp. vanilla concentrate
- 1 tsp. red nourishment shading

Bearings

1. Filter the coconut flour, cocoa powder, salt and preparing pop, and blend.
2. Blend the eggs, erythritol, vanilla, coconut oil, coconut milk, and red nourishment shading. Include them into the dry fixings and blend once more.
3. Separate the hitter between the molds in the doughnut plate. Heat in a preheated stove at 335°F for 16-18 minutes.
4. Expel the doughnuts from the plate and cool for 10 minutes.
5. In a dish, heat the coconut oil to its smoking point and fry the doughnuts on both sides. Channel them in a paper towel.
6. Join the spread, cream cheddar, overwhelming cream, vanilla, and powdered erythritol, beating until it has a feathery consistency. Include the nourishment shading, blend once more, and ice the doughnuts.

Nutrition Info Per Serving

- Calories: 150
- Fat: 15g
- Net Carbs: 2g
- Protein: 2g

COCOA FAT BOMBS

Planning time: 10minutes Cooking time: 0 minutes Serves: 20

Ingrediens:

- 1 cup mascarpone cheddar or full-fat cream cheddar
- ¼ cup grass-nourished spread or additional virgin coconut oil
- 2 tablespoons MCT oil or more coconut oil
- 2 tablespoons crude cocoa powder, unsweetened

- ¼ cup Erythritol or Swerve, powdered
- 10-15 drops fluid Stevia extricate
- ½ teaspoons moment espresso
- 1 teaspoon rum concentrate

INTRUCTIONS:

1. Mellow the mascarpone cheddar and spot in a blender, trailed by the MCT oil, margarine or coconut oil, cocoa powder and sugars.
2. At long last include the moment espresso and heartbeat to arrive at a smooth consistency.
3. Empty the blend into an ice-3D shape plate around 2 tablespoons for each fat bomb.
4. Freeze for around 3 hours until strong.

Nourishment FACTS (PER SERVING) Total Carbohydrates:

- 1g Dietary
- Fiber: 0g
- Net Cabs: 1g
- Protein: 1g

- Absolute Fat: 8g
- Calories: 77

CREAMY COCONUT TRUFFLES

Planning time: 45 minutes Cooking time: 0 minutes Serves: 6

Ingredients:

- ⅓ cup chocolate protein powder
- 2 tablespoons coconut flour
- 2 tablespoons coconut, finely destroyed
- 4 tablespoons canned coconut milk
- 1 tablespoon dull cocoa powder
- 1 tablespoon sugar free smaller than normal chocolate chips
- ⅔ cup coconut spread, relaxed (for covering)
- 1 teaspoon coconut oil, mellowed (for covering)

Direction:

1. Spot the coconut flour, coconut milk, cocoa powder, destroyed coconut, protein powder and chocolate contributes a medium bowl and blend well to join.
2. Delicately spoon the blend into a medium size shape and move to the cooler for 30 minutes.
3. To set up the covering: In a little bowl, join the coconut margarine furthermore, coconut oil. Liquefy in the microwave and mix until smooth.
4. Equitably cover the truffles with the covering blend and spot once more into the refrigerator. Let them refrigerate for another 15-20 minutes.

Nutritional Facts (Per Serving)

- Total Carbohydrates: 2g Dietary
- Fiber: 1g

- Net Cabs: 1g
- Protein: 5g
- All out Fat: 26g
- Calories: 249

TASTY PIZZA FAT BOMBS

Planning time: 20 minutes Cooking time: 0 minutes Serves: 6

Fixings:

- 4 ounces cream cheddar
- 14 cuts Pepperoni
- 8 pitted dark olives
- 2 tablespoons sun dried tomato pesto
- 2 tablespoons crisp basil, hacked
- Salt and pepper to taste

Instructions:

1. In a little bowl, join the tomato pesto, cream cheddar and basil.
2. Meagerly cut the olives and pepperoni and add to the bowl. Blend well to join.
3. Shape the blend into little balls and spot on a serving plate. Chill for 15 minutes and serve decorated with basil leaves and olive.

Nutritional Facts (Per Serving)

- Total Carbohydrates: 2g Dietary
- Fiber: 0g
- Net Cabs: 2g
- Protein: 2g
- All out Fat: 11g
- Calories: 110

LEMON COCONUT FAT BOMBS

Planning time: 5 minutes Cooking time: 0 minutes Serves: 16

Fixings:

- 7 ounces coconut margarine, mellowed
- ¼ cup additional virgin coconut oil, relaxed
- Crisp lemon pizzazz from 1-2 lemons
- 15-20 drops Stevia separate or other sugar to taste
- A touch of salt

Ingredients:

1. Altogether wash the lemons and get-up-and-go them utilizing a fine grater.
2. In a little bowl, mellow the coconut oil and coconut spread. Include the sugar, touch of salt and lemon get-up-and-go. Blend well to join. Drop about 1 tablespoon of coconut blend into a silicone sweet shape or treat paper liners and freeze for an hour until they solidified.
3. Store the done confections in the refrigerator.

Nourishment FACTS (PER SERVING)

- Total Carbohydrates: 3g Dietary
- Fiber: 2
- Net Cabs: 1g
- Protein: 1g
- Complete Fat: 12g
- Calories: 58

CHEDDAR SCRAMBLED EGGS WITH SPINACH

This morning meal gives all of you the supplements expected to begin an awesome day. Green never tasted so great! SERVES 1

INGREDIENTS

- 4 cup new spinach
- 4 eggs
- ½ cup cheddar
- 1 tbsp. substantial cream
- 1 tbsp. olive oil Salt and pepper

Directions

1. In a bowl, combine the eggs, overwhelming cream, salt and pepper.
2. Warmth a huge skillet, and include the olive oil and spinach when the oil is warmed.
3. Mix the spinach, and include the salt and pepper.
4. When the spinach is genuinely shriveled, include the egg blend and go to medium heat.
5. At the point when the eggs are set, include the cheddar and mix gradually until it softens. **Dietary Info Per Serving**

- Calories: 700
- Fat: 58g Net
- Carbs: 5g
- Protein: 43g

BROWNIE MUFFINS FOR KETO HEADS

These biscuits seem as though chocolate however they aren't! Also, why would that be something to be thankful for? Since you can eat them indecently. Made with healthy fixings, they are ideal for an ordinary breakfast. SERVES 6

INGREDIENTS

- 1 cup brilliant flaxseed supper
- 1 tbsp. cinnamon
- ¼ cup cocoa powder
- ½ tsp. salt
- ½ tsp. heating powder
- 1 egg
- 2 tbsp. coconut oil
- ¼ cup sans sugar caramel syrup
- ½ cup pumpkin purée
- 1 tbsp. vanilla concentrate ☐ 1 tbsp. apple juice vinegar
- ¼ cup fragmented almonds

Ingredients

1. Preheat broiler to 350°F.
2. Spot all the fixings aside from the almonds into a huge blending bowl, and join well.
3. In a lined biscuit container, occupy each space, separating the hitter into 6 sections.
4. Sprinkle the almonds on top.
5. Heat for around 15 minutes.

Nutritional Info Per Serving

-
-

Calories: 185

Fat: 13.5g
- Net Carbs: 3.5g
- Protein: 7.4g

KETO CHEDDAR AND SAGE WAFFLE

Waffles are acceptable with syrup, and stunningly better exquisite! Give this choice a shot as a sandwich, or with a cheddar sauce, guacamole, or sauce. SERVES 12

Fixings

- 1 ⅓ cups coconut flour
- 3 tbsp. heating powder
- 1 tsp. ground wise, dried
- ½ tsp. salt
- ¼ tsp. garlic powder
- 2 cups canned coconut milk
- ½ cup water
- 2 eggs
- 3 tbsp. coconut oil, liquefied
- 1 cup cheddar, destroyed

Directions

1. Blend the flour, heating powder and seasonings together in a bowl.
2. Include the coconut milk, water and coconut oil and beat them until they structure a hardened hitter.
3. Join with the cheddar.
4. Oil and warmth the waffle iron, and pour onto each iron area ⅓ cup of the hitter.
5. Close the iron until the waffles are sautéed.

Calories: 214

Fat: 17.2g

- Net Carbs: 3.8g
- Protein: 6.5g

KETO CASSEROLE FOR BREAKFAST

Nutritional Info Per Serving

☐

☐

Dishes are celebrated for being simple – this one is no exemption.

SERVES: 8

INGREDIENTS

- ¼ cup flaxseed dinner
- 1 cup almond flour
- 10 eggs
- 1 lb. breakfast hotdog
- 4 oz. cheddar
- 6 tbsp. light maple syrup
- 4 tbsp. spread
- ½ tsp. onion powder
- ½ tsp. garlic powder
- ¼ tsp. sage
- Salt and pepper

Instructions

1. In a dish on medium warmth, include the morning meal wiener, blending every now and again, until sautéed.
2. In a bowl, blend the flaxseed, almond flour, onion powder, garlic powder and sage together.
3. Add the eggs and cheddar to the bowl, and blend.
4. Add this blend to the hotdog.
5. Line a meal dish with material paper, and pour in the meal blend. Shower the 2 tbsp. of syrup on top.

6. Prepare at 350°F for around 45-55 minutes and cool.

Calories: 480

Fat: 41.2g
- Net Carbs: 3g
- Protein: 22.7g

BREAKFAST BURGERS

Nutritional Info Per Serving

□

□

For the individuals who like an overwhelming breakfast, this is an incredible choice. Joining sweet what's more, flavorful, it's a remarkable choice that you're certain to appreciate. SERVES: 2

INGREDIENTS

- 4 oz. hotdog
- 2 oz. pepper jack cheddar 4 cuts bacon
- 2 eggs
- 1 tbsp. spread
- 1 tbsp. nutty spread powder Salt and pepper

Instructions

1. Prepare the bacon on a cooking sheet at 400°F for 20-25 minutes.
2. Consolidate the margarine and nutty spread powder in a little bowl.
3. Structure 2 patties from the hotdog, and cook them until very much done.
4. Include cheddar, and spread with a cover so it liquefies. Expel from the dish.
5. Cook the egg and set on the burger alongside the nutty spread blend and bacon cuts.

NUTRITIONAL INFO PER SERVING

- Calories: 652
- Fat: 55g

- Net Carbs: 3g
- Protein: 30g

PEANUT BUTTER MUFFINS WITH CHOCOLATE CHIPS

These biscuits are a simple get and-go breakfast. A rich nutty spread flavor – also, a without sugar one, at that – makes certain to dispose of your yearnings. SERVES 2

INGREDIENTS

- ½ cup erythritol
- 1 cup almond flour
- 1 tbsp. preparing powder
- ⅓ cup almond milk
- ⅓ cup nutty spread
- 2 eggs
- ½ cup sans sugar chocolate chips Salt

Directions

1. Blend the erythritol, almond flour, and heating powder in a bowl and whisk.
2. Include the nutty spread and almond milk, and mix.
3. Include the fir st egg and join well. Include the second and join well.
4. Overlap in the chocolate chips.
5. Spot the biscuits in a biscuit tin (of 6 cups) and heat them on 350°F for 15 minutes and cool. **Nourishing Info Per Serving**

- Calories: 527
- Fat: 40g Net
- Carbs: 4.3g

- Protein: 14g

KETO GREEN SMOOTHIE

This wonderful smoothie doesn't have any natural product in it! There's nothing more needed than several minutes to make, and will give you the supplements you have to have an enthusiastic morning. SERVES: 1

INGREDIENTS

- 1½ cups almond milk ☐ 1 oz. spinach
- ⅓ cup cucumber diced
- ⅓ cup celery diced
- ½ cup avocado diced
- 1 tbsp. coconut oil Liquid stevia
- ¼ cup protein powder

Directions

1. Mix the almond milk and spinach in a blender.
2. Prepare for the remainder of the fixings, and mix again until a smooth consistency is accomplished.

NUTRITIONAL INFO PER SERVING

- Calories: 370
- Fat: 24g
- Net Carbs: 5g
- Protein: 27g

KETO OATMEAL

An entire, sound breakfast. You won't have any desire to miss this scrumptious method to treat your body well. Chia seeds are incredible wellspring of solid fats and make an exquisite completing touch.

SERVES: 2

INGREDIENTS

- ¼ cup destroyed coconut, unsweetened, ⅓ cup almonds, chipped, ¼ cup chia seeds, ⅓ cup chipped coconut, unsweetened 1 tsp. unsweetened vanilla concentrate 1 cup hot water ½ cup coconut milk 2 tbsp. erythritol 6-8 drops stevia remove.

Directions

1. In a bowl, place the chipped and destroyed coconut, almonds and chia seeds, putting aside a smidgen of chipped coconut and almond.
2. Include the coconut milk, vanilla concentrate, stevia and join. Include high temp water and let sit for 10-15 minutes.
3. Sprinkle with chipped coconuts and almonds and top with berries (discretionary).

NOURISHING INFO PER SERVING

- Calories: 360
- Fat: 30 g
- Net Carbs: 5 g
- Protein: 9.5 g

CARROT MUFFINS

An ideal keto treat for the fall. The little cheesecake layer is essentially out of this world!

SERVES 9

Ingredients

- On the other hand the Cheesecake Layer: ¾ cup cream cheddar, 1 egg yolk, 2 tbsp. erythritol, 1 tsp. unsweetened vanilla concentrate.
- For the Rest: ½ cup almond flour, 2 tbsp. coconut flour, 1 tbsp. ground chia seeds, ¼ cup Erythritol, 2 tsp. sans gluten preparing powder, 1 tsp. every cinnamon, vanilla powder and ground ginger ⅛ tsp. each ground allspice and nutmeg ½ cup cleaved walnuts 5 egg whites ⅓ cup virgin coconut oil, liquefied ¾ cup carrots, ground 20 drops fluid stevia Liquefied coconut oil for lubing Salt.

Instruction

1. Make the cheesecake layer by combining the cream cheddar, egg yolk, erythritol and vanilla powder.
2. In a different bowl, join well all dry fixings (aside from the walnuts).
3. In an enormous bowl, place the 4 egg yolks and the egg white leftover from the cheesecake layer in a bowl, alongside the liquefied coconut oil and stevia. Blend all things considered, at that point include the dry blend gradually while blending great.
4. In another bowl, beat 4 egg whites until firm pinnacles structure.
5. Delicately blend in with the player ¼ of the egg whites. At that point, cautiously overlay in the rest with a spatula. Include the carrot and walnuts, attempting to keep the hitter as breezy as conceivable.
6. Line a biscuit tin with 9 biscuit paper cups and spoon in the hitter. Top each of them with a piling tbsp. of the cheesecake

blend. Prepare for 30-35 minutes to 320°F. Expel and cool.

Nutritional INFO PER SERVING

- Calories: 270
- Fat: 26g
- Net Carbs: 3.7g
- Protein: 7g

KETO BANANA PANCAKE

This current one's for the entire family. It's similarly as tasty in the first part of the day as it is postworkout.

SERVING SIZE 4

INGREDIENTS

- 2 eggs, 1 banana, 2 tbsp. cashew nuts, ground, ¼ tsp. cinnamon, ¼ tsp. ground cloves 1 tbsp. additional virgin coconut oil
- For the Topping: 3 tbsp. coconut cream ¼ tsp. cinnamon

Instructions

1. Whisk the eggs in a little bowl.
2. In another bowl, pound the bananas with cinnamon, ground cashew nuts and ground cloves. Add the eggs to the blend and join well.
3. Oil a skillet, warmth, and make the hotcakes by pouring enough hitter to make a hand-size flapjack. Flip when the edges are carmelized and the top starts to bubble.
4. At the point when cooked, expel and top with the coconut cream and cinnamon.

NOURISHING INFO PER SERVING

- Calories: 585
- Fat: 45g
- Net Carbs: 27g
- Protein: 20g

KETO FRENCH TOAST

The Keto diet doesn't mean you can't entertain yourself once with some time. This is your opportunity to do only that, directly here. SERVES: 2 portions **Ingredients**

- 14 eggs, isolated 1 cup whey protein, 4 oz. cream cheddar, mollified, 1 cup unsweetened almond milk, 1 tsp. vanilla, 1 tsp. cinnamon, ½ cup spread, ½ cup Granulated sugar of your decision

Instructions

1. Make the bread by blending 12 egg whites for around 10 minutes, or until solid tops structure. Include whey protein mixing tenderly, and overlay in the cream cheddar.
2. Oil two bread dish and pour the player in them. Heat for around 40-45 minutes at 325°F. Expel and let them cool. Cut them to wanted thickness after they have cooled totally.
3. Consolidate 2 eggs in a bowl, ½ cup unsweetened almond milk, vanilla and cinnamon. Dunk the bread cuts in the blend.
4. Spot the bread onto a skillet and flame broil until gently cooked on the two sides. Rehash with the rest.
5. Make the sauce: place the spread in a pan in high warmth. With regards to a bubble, and starts to dark-colored, include the sugar and the other ½ cup almond milk to the dish. Mix rapidly to consolidate, at that point let cool in the search for gold couple minutes before filling a beneficiary. Top the toast with it.

DIETARY INFO PER SERVING

- Calories: 125
- Fat: 15gNet Carbs: 0.7g
- Protein: 6.5g

LITTLE RED CHOCOLATE CAKES

Mug cakes are very well known, and excessively basic. Attempt this scrumptious minimal number today. SERVES: 1

INGREDIENTS

- 1 tbsp. coconut flour, ⅓ cup almond flour, 1 tbsp. beetroot powder, 1 tbsp. unsweetened cocoa powder ¼ tsp. preparing pop 3 tbsp. erythritol ¼ tsp. vanilla powder ¼ cup sharp cream 2 eggs 2 tbsp. additional virgin coconut oil For the Frosting: 2 tbsp. spread, room temperature ¼ cup cream cheddar 1 tbsp. powdered erythritol ¼ tsp. vanilla powder

Instructions

1. In a bowl, blend the almond flour, coconut flour, cacao powder, beetroot powder, heating pop, erythritol and vanilla powder.
2. Include the eggs, liquefied coconut oil and harsh cream, and join well.
3. Spot the blend into two mugs. Microwave every one of them on high for 70-90 seconds.
4. In the interim, set up the icing by blending the spread, erythritol, cream cheddar what's more, vanilla.
5. Ice the completed mug cakes and appreciate it. **Nutritional**

INFO PER SERVING

- Calories: 560
- Fat: 55g
- Net Carbs: 8g
- Protein: 15g

CALIFORNIA STYLE OMELET

New ingredients take this omelet to the following level, and with eggs, bacon and chicken incorporated it's a protein powerhouse. SERVES: 1

INGREDIENTS

- 2 eggs 2 bacon cuts, cooked and hacked 1 oz. shop cut chicken ¼ avocado 1 tomato 1 tbsp. mayonnaise 1 tbsp. mustard

DIRECTIONS

1. Beat the eggs and fill a hot dish. Start to scramble and season.
2. At the point when eggs are mostly cooked, include the chicken, bacon, cut avocado, and tomato.
3. Consolidate the mayo and mustard too and sprinkle inside.
4. Overlay the omelet. Cook for 5 minutes or until warmed through.

DIETARY INFO PER SERVING

- Calories: 417
- Fat: 35g
- Net Carbs: 5g
- Protein: 27g

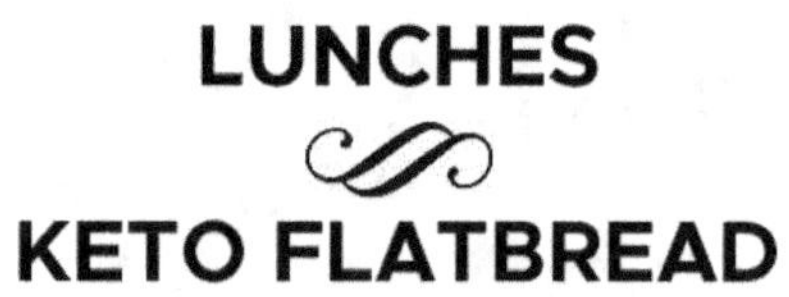

LUNCHES

KETO FLATBREAD

An exemplary formula that will turn out to be a piece of your go-to snacks. This simple formula has apples, ham, and onions – a delightful pizza style mix that you have to attempt! SERVES: 8

INGREDIENTS

For the Crust: 2 cups cream ground mozzarella cheddar, 2 tbsp. cream cheddar ¾ cup almond flour ½ tsp. ocean salt ⅛ tsp. dried thyme.

For the Topping: 1 cup ground Mexican cheddar ½ red onion, little and cut 4 oz. low starch cut ham, cut ¼ medium apple, unpeeled and cut ⅛ tsp. thyme, dried Salt and pepper

DIRECTIONS

1. Fill a pot with a little water and bring to the bubble, at that point turn the warmth to low. Spot the pan inside a metal blending bowl to frame a twofold kettle, and include the mozzarella cheddar, cream cheddar, almond flour, thyme and salt. Mix with a spatula.

2. Cook until the cheddar melts, and blend the ingredients into a mixture. Pour a few onto a 12-inch pizza plate secured with material paper. Fold the mixture into a ball and spot onto the focal point of the material paper. Pat into a circle shape to spread the skillet.

3. Spot the mixture and the material paper on the pizza dish, jabbing openings all through the mixture with a fork, and prepare for 6-8 minutes at 425°F. Evacuate.

4. Spread the garnishes over the flatbread, alongside the cheddar, onion, apple furthermore, the ham. Spread with more cheddar. Season with thyme, salt and pepper.

5. Heat again at 350°F for 5-7 minutes. Expel once the cheddar starts to darker. Let cool before cutting.

NUTRITIONAL INFO PER SERVING

- Calories: 257
- Fat: 22g
- Net Carbs: 5g
- Protein: 18g

ZUCCHINI BOATS

This stuffed zucchini is a stunning alternative for a quick and delectable lunch pressed with protein. SERVES 1

INGREDIENTS

- 2 enormous zucchini, 2 tbsp. spread, 3 oz. destroyed cheddar, 1 cup broccoli, 6 oz. destroyed rotisserie chicken, 1 stalk green onion, 2 tbsp. harsh cream Salt and pepper.

DIRECTIONS

1. Cut the zucchini down the middle the long way, scooping out the center until you are left with a pontoon shape.
2. Into every zucchini pour a little dissolved margarine, season, and spot into the broiler at 400°F, preparing for around 18 minutes.
3. In a bowl, consolidate the chicken, broccoli, and acrid cream.
4. Spot the chicken blend inside the emptied zucchinis.
5. Top with cheddar and prepare for an extra 10-15 minutes.

NUTRITIONAL INFO PER SERVING

- Calories: 480
- Fat: 35g
- Net Carbs: 5g
- Protein: 28g

KETO STROMBOLI

Stromboli is a conventional Italian formula that takes after collapsed pizza. This keto ham and cheddar adaptation make certain to please.
SERVES: 4

INGREDIENTS

- 1¼ cup destroyed mozzarella cheddar 4 tbsp. Almond flour 3 tbsp. Coconut flour 1 egg 1 tsp. Italian flavoring 4 oz. Ham 4 oz. cheddar Salt and pepper

DIRECTIONS

1. Soften the mozzarella cheddar in the microwave for around 1 moment, blending once in a while so as not to consume it.
2. In a different bowl, blend almond flour, coconut flour, salt, and pepper and include the softened mozzarella cheddar. Blend well. At that point, in the wake of letting it chill off a piece, include the eggs and join once more.
3. Spot the blend on material paper, laying a subsequent layer on top. Utilizing your hands or moving pin, level it out into a square shape.
4. Expel the top layer of paper and with a blade cut corner to corner lines toward the center of the batter. They ought to be cut ⅓ of the path in on one side. At that point, cut corner to corner lines on the opposite side as well.
5. On the highest point of the batter, exchange cuts of ham and cheddar. At that point, overlay one side over, and afterward the other, to cover the filling.
6. Spot on a preparing sheet and heat at 400°F for 15-20 minutes.

DIETARY INFO PER SERVING

- Calories: 305
- Fat: 22g
- Net Carbs: 5g

- Protein: 25g

KETO CHICKEN SANDWICH

Make plain keto cloud bread into an extravagant chicken sandwich. Bacon and avocado make it considerably increasingly brilliant. SERVES 2

INGREDIENTS

- For the Bread: 3 eggs, 3 oz. cream cheddar, ⅛ tsp. cream of tartar Salt Garlic powder
- For the Filling: 1 tbsp. mayonnaise, 1 tsp. sriracha, 2 cuts bacon, 3 oz. chicken, 2 cuts pepper jack cheddar, 2 grape tomatoes, ¼ avocado.

DIRECTIONS

1. Separate the eggs in various dishes. In the egg whites include cream tartar, salt what's more, beat until hardened pinnacles structure.
2. In another bowl, beat the egg yolks with cream cheddar. Consolidate the blend into the egg white blend and join cautiously.
3. Spot the player on a material paper and structure minimal square shapes that look like bread cuts. Shimmer garlic powder on top and heat at 300°F for 25 minutes.
4. While the bread is heating, cook the chicken and bacon in a griddle, flavoring to taste.
5. At the point when the bread is done, expel from broiler and let cool for 10-15 minutes.

At that point, make the sandwich with the cooked chicken and bacon, including the mayo, sriracha, tomatoes, cheddar and crushed avocado to taste.

DIETARY INFO PER SERVING

- Calories: 360
- Fat: 28g
- Net Carbs: 3g
- Protein: 22g

FISH BITES WITH AVOCADO

This is one of a kind fish nibbles that can be served close by a new plate of mixed greens. The avocado packs a fabulous Omega 3 fat punch!

SERVES: 8

INGREDIENTS

- 10 oz. depleted canned fish ¼ cup mayo 1 avocado ¼ cup parmesan cheddar ⅓ cup almond flour ½ tsp. garlic powder ¼ tsp. onion powder ½ cup coconut oil Salt and pepper

DIRECTIONS

1. In a bowl blend all the ingredients (except for coconut oil). Structure little balls and spread with almond flour.
2. Fry them in a skillet medium warmth with dissolved coconut oil (it must be hot) until they appear to be caramelized on all sides.

Nutritional INFO PER SERVING

- Calories: 137
- Fat: 12g
- Net Carbs: 10g
- Protein: 6g

KETO GREEN SALAD

Who said the green serving of mixed greens must be dull? These ingredients and the great dressing will fill your heart with joy. SERVES 1

INGREDIENTS

- 2 oz. blended greens 3 tbsp. simmered pine nuts 2 tbsp. raspberry vinaigrette 2 tbsp. parmesan, shaved 2 cuts bacon Salt and pepper

DIRECTIONS

1. Cook the bacon in a skillet until crunchy and all around sautéed. Separate into pieces, and add to the remainder of the ingredients in a bowl.
2. Dress the serving of mixed greens with the raspberry vinaigrette.

Nutritional INFO PER SERVING

- Calories: 480
- Fat: 37g
- Net Carbs: 4g
- Protein: 17g

ORIGINAL KETO STUFFED HOT DOGS

Have only 10 minutes for lunch? No stresses, this unique formula is here to help you out! SERVES: 6

INGREDIENTS

- 6 franks 12 cuts bacon 2 oz. cheddar ½ tsp. cheddar garlic powder ½ tsp. onion powder Salt and pepper

DIRECTIONS

1. Make a little cut in each frank, and stuff them with cuts of cheddar. Wrap each sausage with 2 cuts of covering bacon, and secure with toothpicks.
2. Over a wire rack (with a treat sheet underneath), place the sausages. Season them and prepare at 400°F for 20-25 minutes approx.

NUTRITONAL INFO PER SERVING

- Calories: 385
- Fat: 34g
- Net Carbs: 0.5g
- Protein: 17g

EASY EGG SOUP

5 minutes and 5 ingredients can make enchantment stuff—like this yummy egg soup. SERVES 1

INGREDIENTS

- 1½ cups chicken juices, ½ solid shape of chicken bouillon, 1 tbsp. bacon fat, 2 eggs, 1 tsp. bean stew garlic glue.

DIRECTIONS

1. In a skillet on the stove on a medium-high warmth, include the chicken juices, bouillon shape and bacon fat. Bring into a bubble and join bean stew garlic glue and blend.

2. Whisk the eggs and add them to the chicken while blending, at that point let sit for a few moments.

NUTRITIONAL INFO PER SERVING

- Calories: 280
- Fat: 25g
- Net Carbs: 2.7g
- Protein: 13g

KETO SAUSAGE AND PEPPER SOUP

A flavorful low-carb soup that will execute your craving dead and keep out the virus. SERVES: 6

INGREDIENTS

- 30 oz. pork frankfurter 1 tbsp. olive oil 10 oz. crude spinach 1 medium green ringer pepper 1 can tomatoes with jalapeños 4 cups hamburger stock 1 tbsp. onion powder 1 tbsp. bean stew powder 1 tsp. cumin garlic powder 1 tsp. Italian flavoring Salt

DIRECTIONS

1. In a huge pot, heat the olive oil over medium warmth until hot and cook the hotdog. Mix.
2. Hack the green pepper and add to the pot. Mix well. Season with salt and pepper include the tomatoes and jalapeños. Mix.
3. Include the spinach top and spread the pot. At the point when it is shriveled, fuse flavors and juices and join.
4. Spread the pot again and let cook for around 30 minutes (heat medium-low).

At the point when it is done, evacuate the top and let the soup stew for around 10 minutes.

Dietary INFO PER SERVING

- Calories: 525
- Fat: 45g
- Net Carbs: 4g
- Protein: 28g

MUG CAKE WITH JALAPEÑO

Feeling hot, hot, hot? In the event that you like jalapeño peppers, you'll revere this unique mug cake. SERVES 1

INGREDIENTS

- 2 tbsp. almond flour
- 1 tbsp. flaxseed dinner
- 1 tbsp. spread
- 1 tbsp. cream cheddar
- 1 egg
- 1 bacon cut, cooked
- ½ jalapeño pepper, cut
- ½ tsp. preparing powder
- ¼ tsp. salt

DIRECTIONS

1. Cook the bacon on a medium warmth in a skillet until firm.
2. Blend all the ingredients in a compartment and pour some inside a mug. Microwave for 75 seconds on high.
3. Cautiously take out the mug cake out and let cool before eating.

DIETARY INFO PER SERVING

- Calories: 430
- Fat: 40g
- Net Carbs: 4g
- Protein: 17g

NEW KETO SANDWICH

Make this new sandwich with ingredients effectively found in your ice chest. Put intoyour Tupperware, spread, and go! SERVES 1

INGREDIENTS

- 1 cucumber 1 ½ oz. boursin cheddar Meat of your decision, cut

DIRECTIONS

1. Cut the cucumber down the middle and scoop out the center and seeds with a spoon. Expel the hard external skin cautiously with a blade.
2. In one side spot cheddar. In the opposite side overlay meat. Spot together to shape a sandwich!

DIETARY INFO PER SERVING

- Calories: 195
- Fat: 14g
- Net Carbs: 8g
- Protein: 18g

ORIGINAL SQUASH LASAGNA

You've likely utilized spaghetti squash to make spaghetti. Be that as it may, have you attempted it for lasagna? SERVES 12

INGREDIENTS

- 1 lb. spaghetti squash, 3 lb. ground meat, 30 cuts mozzarella cheddar, 1 huge container marinara sauce, 32 oz. entire milk ricotta cheddar.

DIRECTIONS

1. Cut the spaghetti squash in two parts, putting them face down onto a preparing dish. Include a half inch or so of water. Prepare for 45 minutes. At the point when wrapped up, cautiously pull out the meat of the squash.
2. In a griddle, cook the ground hamburger the meat in a dish and include marinara sauce.
3. In a lubed heating dish, place a layer of spaghetti squash, spread with the meat sauce, mozzarella and ricotta. Rehash until the skillet is full.
4. Heat for 35 minutes at 375°F.

NOURISHING INFO PER SERVING

- Calories: 710
- Fat: 60g
- Net Carbs: 17g
- Protein: 45g

CHILI SOUP

Utilize your slow cooker to make this yummy soup, ideal for a crisp day. Get it? Great. SERVES: 8

INGREDIENTS

- 2 tbsp. spread unsalted, 2 onions, 1 pepper, 8 chicken thighs (boneless) 8 cuts of bacon, 1 tsp. thyme, 1 tsp. salt 1 tsp. pepper, 1 tbsp. garlic, minced, 1 tbsp. coconut flour 3 tbsp. lemon juice 1 cup chicken stock ¼ cup unsweetened, coconut milk 3 tbsp. tomato glue

DIRECTIONS

1. Spot the spread in the focal point of the CrockPot.
2. Cut the onion and pepper, and add to the CrockPot. At that point include the chicken thighs. Top with the bacon cuts.
3. Season with salt, pepper, minced garlic, and coconut flour. Include the lemon juice, chicken stocks, coconut milk and tomato glue.
4. Cook on low for 6 hours. At the point when it is done, mix and serve.

NOURISHING INFO PER SERVING

- Calories: 395
- Fat: 20g
- Net Carbs: 8g
- Protein: 40g

CHICKEN NUGGETS FOR KETO NUTS

These are brisk and more beneficial than any pieces you'll ever pay off the rack! Attempt them and see with your own eyes. SERVES: 4

INGREDIENTS

- 1 chicken bosom, precooked, ½ ounce ground parmesan, 2 tbsp. almond flour, ½ tsp. preparing powder, 1 egg, 1 tbsp. water.

DIRECTIONS

1. Cut the chicken bosom into cuts and afterward into scaleddown pieces. Put in a safe spot.
2. Consolidate the parmesan, almond flour, preparing powder, and water. Mix.
3. Spread the chicken pieces into the hitter, and afterward place straightforwardly into the hot oil. Evacuate when brilliant.

NUTRITIONAL INFO PER SERVING

- Calories: 165
- Fat: 9g
- Net Carbs: 3g
- Protein: 25g

CAULIFLOWER RICE WITH CHICKEN

Riced cauliflower is a decent choice when you need to cook for many individuals. Likewise, it is low-carb, and when joined with curry chicken, you'll have an extraordinary wellspring of protein. SERVES 6

INGREDIENTS

- 4 chicken bosoms
- 1 parcel curry glue
- 1 cup water
- 3 tbsp. ghee

- ½ cup substantial cream
- 1 head cauliflower

DIRECTIONS

1. In an enormous container, dissolve the ghee, include the curry, and mix. At the point when consolidated, include the water, and stew for 5 minutes.

2. Include the chicken, spread and continue cooking for 20 minutes more. At the point when it is done, include the cream and cook for 5 extra minutes.

3. Independently, set up the cauliflower rice: slash the head into florets and shred. Sauté in a griddle with a little margarine or olive oil, and afterward go to low, covering with a top. Let it steam for 5-8 minutes.

4. Serve alongside the chicken curry.

NUTRITIONAL INFO PER SERVING

- Calories: 350
- Fat: 16g
- Net Carbs: 10g
- Protein: 40g

ZUCCHINI KETO WRAPS

This one must be attempted to be accepted. It serves up to 6 and the blend of goat's cheddar, mint and dill give it an absolutely exceptional contort. SERVES: 6

INGREDIENTS

- 1 zucchini 6 oz. delicate goat's cheddar 1 tbsp. dried mint 1 tsp. dried dill Salt and pepper Oil

DIRECTIONS

1. Remove the parts of the bargains. Cut into ⅛ - inch cuts and brush with oil. Flame broil on the two sides.
2. Combine the goat's cheddar, mint and dill. Separation into 6 pieces.
3. Wrap the cheddar pieces with the zucchini cuts and secure with a toothpick.

DIETARY INFO PER SERVING

- Calories: 188
- Fat: 14g
- Net Carbs: 4g
- Protein: 15g

CAULIFLOWER SOUP WITH BACON AND CHEDDAR

This soup will warm you up on a chilly day. The healthy bacon and cheddar season makes it one that even exacting eaters will eat straight up!

SERVES: 6

INGREDIENTS

- 1 head of cauliflower, 2 tbsp. olive oil, 1 medium onion, diced 4 cuts bacon 1 tbsp. minced garlic 1 tsp. thyme 12 oz. matured cheddar 1 oz. parmesan cheddar 3 cups chicken soup ¼ cup substantial cream.

DIRECTIONS

1. Hack the cauliflower and spot-on a foil-lined heating sheet. Sprinkle olive oil what's more, season it with salt and pepper. Heat for 35 minutes at 375°F.
2. In a pot, cook the bacon until fresh. Include diced onion and fry it in the bacon oil. At the point when it is delicate, include the garlic and the thyme, and cook for 1 moment or less.
3. Consolidate the chicken stock and cauliflower, and stew, secured, for 20 minutes.
4. When time is up, mix the ingredients in a nourishment processor or blender until smooth. Spot over into the pot. Include the cheddar and the parmesan cheddar, and mix until dissolved.
5. At last, include the bacon and the twofold cream, and blend well. If necessary, stew for 10 minutes more, or until warmed.

DIETARY INFO PER SERVING

- Calories: 340
- Fat: 26g
- Net Carbs: 10g
- Protein: 20g

KETO CASSEROLE WITH CHICKEN AND BACON

This dish is a finished dinner: chicken, bacon, hotdog, veggies and cheddar will assist you with remaining loaded with vitality for the remainder of your day. SERVES: 12

INGREDIENTS

- 12 chicken thighs
- 1 little onion
- 4 celery stalks
- 24 oz. Jimmy Dean hotdog
- 16 oz. cut mushrooms
- 16 oz. solidified cauliflower
- 7 cuts bacon
- 8 oz. destroyed cheddar
- 16 oz. cream cheddar, mollified Paprika

DIRECTIONS

1. In the stove, cook the bacon at 400°F for 15 minutes.
2. In the interim, dice the chicken and cook in a skillet. Expel from the dish.
3. Dark-colored the hotdog. When it is done, move it to a similar bowl as the chicken.
4. Hack the onion and celery, and cook them in the rest of the wiener oil until translucent.
5. Defrost the cauliflower, and cut the florets into little pieces.
6. In a huge bowl, include all the ingredients and blend well. Include the cream cheddar also, blend well.

7. In a huge skillet, place the blend and sprinkle the paprika.

8. Prepare at 350°F for 30 minutes, secured with a foil. Reveal and cook for an extra 10 minutes.

NUTRITIONAL INFO PER SERVING

- Calories: 600
- Fat: 41g
- Net Carbs: 6g
- Protein: 53g

MEXICAN-STYLE CASSEROLE WITH SPINACH

This low-carb dish has all the yummy kind of tacos, however with a more advantageous contort. SERVES: 12

INGREDIENTS

- 1 green pepper
- 1 onion
- 0 oz. depleted spinach 2 lb. ground pork
- 2 jars depleted diced tomatoes with green chilies
- 10 tbsp. sharp cream
- 8 oz. mozzarella cheddar, destroyed
- 16 oz. cream cheddar
- 4 tsp. taco flavoring Jalapeños, cut

DIRECTIONS

1. Hack pepper and onion and cook them until translucent. Discretionary: include diced jalapeños.
2. Spot the pepper and onion into a bowl.
3. Cook the spinach by shrinking it in a griddle with a little olive oil. At the point when it is done, add it to the bowl.
4. Cook the ground pork until sautéed. Season with taco flavoring.
5. Add the diced tomato to the bowl, and consolidate the harsh cream, mozzarella what's more, cream cheddar. Empty the blend into a heating dish, and prepare at 350°F for 40 minutes.

NUTRITIONAL INFO PER SERVING

- Calories: 400
- Fat: 30g

- Net Carbs: 10g
- Protein: 25g

ALMOND PIZZA

Pizza can be a sound choice when you make the covering with almond dinner. Include your preferred fixings and appreciate. SERVES: 4

INGREDIENTS

- ¾ cup almond supper, 1½ tsp. preparing powder, 1½ tsp. granulated sugar, ½ tsp. oregano, ¼ tsp. thyme, ½ tsp. garlic powder, 2 eggs, 5 tbsp. spread, ½ cup alfredo sauce, 4 oz. cheddar

DIRECTIONS

1. Combine the dry ingredients in a huge bowl.
2. Take the eggs (at room temperature) and add to the dry blend.
3. Dissolve the margarine and fuse.
4. On a lubed pizza dish, spread the covering and pre-cook at 350°F for around 7 minutes.
5. Expel from the stove, and spread the Alfredo Sauce and cheddar on top. Let cook for 5 minutes more.

Dietary INFO PER SERVING

- Calories: 460
- Fat: 45g
- Net Carbs: 5g
- Protein: 15g

CRAB STUFFED MUSHROOMS WITH BACON

Makes 5 Servings

Readiness: 20 min , Cook Time: 30 min The Ketosis Cookbook

Tidbits and Dips Per Serving - Fat: 24g Protein: 23g Net Carbs: 8g 1 pound . enormous mushrooms (around 20) – cleaned and destemmed 12 ounces crab meat 6 strips bacon – cooked fresh and disintegrated 6m ounces cream cheddar – mellowed 1/3 cup sharp cheddar – destroyed 1/4 cup acrid cream 3 cloves garlic – minced, 3 green onions – cleaved, 1 tablespoon Dijon ocean salt and pepper – to taste 1/2 cup Parmesan cheddar – destroyed

1. Preheat broiler to 400° Line a rimmed preparing sheet with aluminum foil. Prepare mushroom tops for 10 minutes. Spill out any abundance dampness that pools in the tops of the mushrooms. In an enormous blending bowl, consolidate crab, bacon, cream cheddar, cheddar, harsh cream, garlic, green onions, Dijon, salt and pepper. Blend until all ingredients are very much consolidated.

2. Stuff each mushroom with crab blend. Heat for an extra 10 minutes expel from the stove and top each mushroom with Parmesan cheddar. Prepare for 5- 10 minutes or until cheddar on top is brilliant dark-colored.

SUPPERS

MEATBALLS WITH BACON AND CHEESE

Take meatballs to the following level. These are succulent and taste incredible. A particularly great alternative when you have individuals over!

SERVES 5

INGREDIENTS

- 1½ lb. ground hamburger, ¾ cup pork skins, squashed ¾ tsp. salt, ¾ tsp. pepper, ¾ tsp. cumin,¾ tsp. garlic powder ¾ cup cheddar 4 cuts bacon, 1 egg

DIRECTIONS

1. Procedure the pork skins to make a powder.
2. Blend the ground hamburger, pork skins, salt, pepper, cumin and garlic powder. Include the cheddar and blend well.
3. Cut the bacon into little pieces and fry them in a hot skillet until they come to the wanted doneness. Allow them to cool. Add the bacon to the meat and join well.
4. Structure the meatballs.
5. Cook the meatballs in a container, searing them on all sides, at that point spread with a cover for 10 minutes. At the point when completed, let them sit for 5 minutes or so before getting a charge out of. Top with your preferred sauce.

NOURISHING INFO PER SERVING

- Calories: 450
- Fat: 26g
- Net Carbs: 3g
- Protein: 50g

BACON WRAPPED CHICKEN

A basic formula with chicken and bacon, sure to go down as a champ in everybody's book. It's anything but difficult to make it and completely stacked with protein. SERVES: 4

INGREDIENTS

- 2 skinless chicken bosoms, boneless 2 oz. blue cheddar, 4 cuts ham, 8 cuts bacon

DIRECTIONS

1. Cut the bosom parts down the middle longwise.
2. Spread out 2 cuts of ham, and spot a line of cheddar in the center. Move up, and place inside the chicken bosom.
3. Wrap the chicken bosom with 4 cuts of bacon, covering the whole bosom.
4. Spot the bosoms in a broiler verification skillet (lubed with spread or coconut oil); furthermore, dark-colored the bacon everywhere. Expel from the skillet and spot in the broiler to cook for 45 minutes at 325°F. Let sit for 10 minutes before serving.

DIETARY INFO PER SERVING

- Calories: 270
- Fat: 11g
- Net Carbs: 0.50g
- Protein: 38g

KETO BROCCOLI SOUP

You can likely discover all the ingredients for this one in your refrigerator as of now, so thump it up and appreciate! SERVES: 4

INGREDIENTS

- 1 head broccoli, ¼ cup overwhelming cream ¼ cup cream cheddar ¼ cup harsh cream ¼ cup almond milk 4 oz. cheddar ½ onion ½ chicken bouillon 3D shape

DIRECTIONS

1. Expel the florets from the broccoli. Steam them on the stove.
2. Put the florets into a blender and include the remainder of the ingredients. Mix until the blend arrives at the ideal consistency.
3. Fill a pot and stew until warmed (10 minutes or somewhere in the vicinity).

NUTRITIONAL INFO PER SERVING

- Calories: 270
- Fat: 25g
- Net Carbs: 8g
- Protein: 10g

LITTLE PORTOBELLO PIZZA

These little pizzas are produced using Portobello tops. A unique method to complete your day and hold those longings under tight restraints.

SERVES: 1

INGREDIENTS

- 3 Portobello mushrooms Olive oil
- 3 tsp. pizza flavoring 3 tomato cuts
- 9 spinach leaves
- 1½ oz. mozzarella
- 1½ oz. Monterey jack
- 1½ oz. cheddar 12 pepperoni cuts

DIRECTIONS

1. Set up the Portobello mushrooms by washing them, expelling both the gills what's more, the stems.
2. Sprinkle with olive oil and pizza flavoring, and afterward top with the various ingredients, aside from the pepperoni cuts.
3. Cook at 450°F for 6 minutes. Include the pepperoni cuts and cook until firm.

NOURISHING INFO PER SERVING

- Calories: 275
- Fat: 20g
- Net Carbs: 5g
- Protein: 20g

BACON WRAP

Flavorful, stuffed with protein and set decent and quick. What's not to love?

SERVES: 4

INGREDIENTS

- 16 oz. hamburger Montreal steak flavoring 4 bacon cuts

DIRECTIONS

1. Cut the hamburger into 3D shapes and season it.
2. Cut the bacon cuts in four.
3. Wrap the hamburger with the bacon, and puncture with a toothpick. Rehash 2 or 3 times. Fry for 3 minutes.

NUTRITIONAL INFO PER SERVING

- Calories: 217
- Fat: 10g
- Net Carbs: 0g
- Protein: 30g

CHEDDAR BISCUITS

We love our cheddar bread rolls. Stuff them with your preferred fillings, or have them as a side to your preferred supper dish. SERVES: 1

INGREDIENTS

- 2 cups Carbquik 2 oz. unsalted spread, cold 4 oz. destroyed cheddar ½ tsp. garlic powder ½ tsp. salt ¼ cup substantial cream ¼ cup water

DIRECTIONS

1. In a bowl, blend Carbquik and include the virus margarine. Cut in the bits of spread until the blend has little chunks of spread and flour about the size of peas. Include the cheddar, garlic powder and salt and join together.

2. Include substantial cream and water. Blend until a batter structure. Separate them into 6 pieces and spot on a lubed sheet. Heat them at 450°F for around 8-10 minutes.

DIETARY INFO PER SERVING

- Calories: 45
- Fat: 4g
- Net Carbs: 2.5g
- Protein: 1.6g

SAUSAGE AND CABBAGE SKILLET MELT

Somewhat hot, too fulfilling and ideal for a keto supper. Give this one a shot with organization. SERVES 4

INGREDIENTS

- 4 zesty Italian chicken wieners 1½ cups green cabbage, destroyed 1½ cups purple cabbage, destroyed ½ cup onion, diced 2 tsp. coconut oil 2 cuts Colby jack cheddar 2 tsp. crisp cilantro, cleaved

DIRECTIONS

1. Shred the cabbage (or use pre-destroyed cabbage) and cleave the onion.
2. Liquefy the coconut oil, and fry the onion and cabbage in a huge skillet. Go to medium-high and cook for 8 minutes.
3. Include the wiener, and mix to blend it into the vegetables. Cook for 8 further minutes.
4. Include the cheddar top and spread.

5. Mood killer the warmth and pause while the cheddar liquefies into the vegetables.

Nourishing INFO PER SERVING

- Calories: 233
- Fat: 15g
- Net Carbs: 5g
- Protein: 20g

KETO CHICKEN TIKKA MASALA

Chicken Tikka Masala is a too delightful and delectable curry that you can now make keto style! SERVES 5

INGREDIENTS

- 1 lb. chicken thighs (boneless/skinless) 2 tbsp. olive oil 2 tsp. onion powder 3 minced garlic cloves 1 inch ground ginger root 3 tbsp. tomato glue 5 tsp. garam masala 2 tsp. smoked paprika 4 tsp. fit salt 10 oz. diced tomatoes (can) 1 cup substantial cream 1 cup coconut milk, Crisp cleaved cilantro, 1 tsp. guar gum

DIRECTIONS

1. De-bone the chicken thighs. Slash the chicken into reduced down pieces.
2. In a moderate cooker, include the chicken and mesh the ginger on top.
3. In another bowl, blend the tomato glue and canned tomatoes with the remainder of the dry flavors. Include ½ cup coconut milk and mix. Add to the moderate cooker.
4. Cook on low for 6 hours or on high for 3 hours.

5. When completed, include the rest of the coconut milk, twofold cream, and guar gum. Blend.

NUTRITIONAL INFO PER SERVING

- Calories: 495
- Fat: 43g
- Net Carbs: 5g
- Protein: 25g Sweets

AMARETTI COOKIES

These treats are anything but difficult to make and can bolster a little swarm. Or then again only you, for a couple days! SERVES: 16 treats

INGREDIENTS

- 1 cup almond flour
- 2 tbsp. coconut flour ½ tsp. preparing powder
- ¼ tsp. cinnamon
- ½ tsp. salt
- ½ cup erythritol
- 2 eggs
- 4 tbsp. coconut oil
- ½ tsp. vanilla concentrate
- ½ tsp. almond remove 2 tbsp. without sugar jam 1 tbsp. coconut, destroyed

DIRECTIONS

1. Join all the dry ingredients.
2. Include the wet ingredients. Blend well.

3. In a material paper lined on a heating sheet, structure the treats. Make a gouge in every single one of them. Heat at 400°F for around 16 minutes. Let them cool.

4. Include each indent a smidgen of jam, and top with a sprinkle of destroyed coconut.

DIETARY INFO PER SERVING

- Calories: 86
- Fat: 8g
- Net Carbs: 1g
- Protein: 2.5g

PUMPKIN ICE CREAM WITH PECANS

Two exemplary flavors are joined into one right now, ideal for fall nighttimes.

SERVES 4

INGREDIENTS

- ½ cup toasted and hacked walnuts 2 tbsp. salted spread ½ cup curds ½ cup pumpkin puree 1 tsp. pumpkin flavor 2 cups coconut milk 3 egg yolks ½ tsp. thickener ⅓ cup erythritol 20 drops fluid stevia 1 tsp. maple extricate

DIRECTIONS

1. Broil the margarine and walnuts in a pan for 8-10 minutes.
2. Mix together the remainder of the ingredients utilizing a submersion blender.
3. Add the blend to a frozen yogurt machine, including the walnuts and margarine top.
4. Adhere to the directions of the machine, and appreciate.

NUTRITIONAL INFO PER SERVING

- Calories: 250
- Fat: 22g
- Net Carbs: 4g
- Protein: 7g

PEANUT BUTTER BAR

It's anything but difficult to make, and much simpler to eat – be cautious or you'll build up a nut spread enslavement! SERVES: 8

INGREDIENTS

- For the Crust: 1 cup almond flour ¼ liquefied cup margarine ½ tsp. cinnamon 1 tbsp. erythritol Salt
- For the Fudge: ¼ cup overwhelming cream ¼ cup liquefied margarine ½ cup nutty spread ¼ cup erythritol ½ tsp. vanilla concentrate ⅛ tsp. thickener For the Topping: ⅓ cup slashed vegetarian dim chocolate

DIRECTIONS

1. Consolidate the almond flour, erythritol, cinnamon and salt with half of the liquefied margarine.
2. Pack the blend into a preparing dish fixed with material paper. Heat for 10 minutes and let cool.
3. Mix the fudge ingredients.
4. Spread the blend over the covering and include the slashed chocolate top.
5. Spot in the cooler and freeze for 1-2 hours.

NUTRITIONAL INFO PER SERVING

- Calories: 300Fat: 20g
- Net Carbs: 3g
- Protein: 5g

STRAWBERRY AND CREAM CAKES

A light, soft cake ideal for a mid-year grill or as a light pastry.

SERVES: 5

INGREDIENTS

- For the Mix: 3 eggs 3 oz. cream cheddar ¼ tsp. preparing powder ½ tsp. vanilla concentrate 2 tbsp. erythritol
- For the Filling: 10 strawberries 1 cup overwhelming cream

DIRECTIONS

1. Separate the eggs. Whisk the egg whites until hardened pinnacles structure. In another bowl, include the egg yolks, the cream cheddar, preparing powder, vanilla concentrate and the erythritol and join until smooth.
2. Delicately consolidate the egg white blend into the egg yolk blend by collapsing. Structure the blend into little cake shapes on a heating sheet secured with material paper.
3. Whip the substantial cream until thick.
4. Heat at 300°F for 25-30 minutes. Allow them to cool. Cut them open and spot strawberries and cream inside.

NUTRITIONAL INFO PER SERVING

- Calories: 275
- Fat: 30g
- Net Carbs: 3.7g
- Protein: 6g

POPPY SEED SOUFFLÉS

These soufflés are low-carb, and the sensitive lemon poppy seed season gives a somewhat unique wind to one of our preferred staples. SERVES 4

INGREDIENTS

- 2 isolated huge eggs
- ¼ cup erythritol
- 1 cup entire milk ricotta 2 tsp. lemon get-up-and-go
- 1 tbsp. lemon juice
- 1 tsp. vanilla concentrate
- 1 tsp. poppy seeds

DIRECTIONS

1. Whisk the egg whites until frothy. Include erythritol and beat until solid pinnacles structure.
2. Blend the egg yolks in with ricotta cheddar and erythritol. Include the lemon get-up-and-go and juice.
3. Fuse the concentrate and poppy seed and blend well.
4. Include the egg white into the blend via cautiously collapsing.
5. Separation the hitter into 4 little ramekins and prepare at 375°F for around 20 minutes. Take care not to open the stove until they are done or they may breakdown.

NOURISHING INFO PER SERVING

- Calories: 150
- Fat: 10g
- Net Carbs: 3g
- Protein: 10g

KETO CHOC TARTS

Chocolate and nutty spread are combined right now keto formula.

SERVES: 4

INGREDIENTS

- For the Crust: ¼ cup flaxseed supper
- 2 tbsp. almond flour
- 1 tbsp. erythritol
- 1 egg white
- For the Top Layer: Avocado
- 4 tbsp. cocoa powder
- ¼ cup erythritol
- ½ tsp. vanilla concentrate ½ tsp. cinnamon
- 2 tbsp. substantial cream
- For the Middle Layer: 4 tbsp. nutty spread 2 tbsp. spread

DIRECTIONS

1. Make the covering by beating the flaxseed until the blend is coarse. Include the rest of the outside layer ingredients and blend well.
2. Spot the outside layer inside tart skillet making a point to squeeze them to the base. Get the sides up. Prepare at 350°F for 8 minutes. Evacuate and let them cool.
3. In a little blender, consolidate all the top layer ingredients until smooth.
4. Dissolve the nutty spread with the margarine in the microwave to make the center layer.
5. Pour the center layer blend onto the tarts and spot in the ice chest for 30 minutes or until it is set. At the point when it is done, include the top layer. Spot in the ice chest for 30 more minutes.

NUTRITIONAL INFO PER SERVING

- Calories: 300
- Fat: 27g
- Net Carbs: 4g
- Protein: 10g

EASY PUMPKIN PIE CHEESECAKE

This yummy cheesecake doesn't have to heat. It's the ideal smooth dessert after a Thanksgiving supper! SERVES 8

INGREDIENTS

For the Crust:

- ¾ cup almond flour
- ½ cup flaxseed supper
- ½ cup margarine
- 1 tsp. pumpkin pie zest
- 25 drops fluid stevia **For the Filling:**

- 4 oz. cream cheddar
- ⅓ cup pumpkin puree
- 2 tbsp. acrid cream
- ¼ cup substantial cream
- 3 tbsp. margarine
- ¼ tsp. pumpkin pie zest
- 25 drops fluid stevia

DIRECTIONS

1. Consolidate all the dry ingredients for the outside and include the margarine and stevia. Blend.
2. Spot some batter into a tart dish and press it to the base.
3. Blend all the filling ingredients and mix with a submersion blender.
4. Empty the filling into coverings and refrigerate for 4 hours. Top with whipped cream whenever wanted.

NOURISHING INFO PER SERVING

- Calories: 267
- Fat: 25g
- Net Carbs: 4g
- Protein: 6g

AVOCADO ICE CREAM WITH CHOCOLATE

This unique avocado frozen yogurt additionally has an energizing chocolate component that will go down a treat with loved ones.

SERVES: 6

INGREDIENTS

- 2 avocados
- 1 cup coconut milk
- ½ cup substantial cream
- ½ cup cocoa powder
- 2 tsp. vanilla concentrate
- ½ cup powdered erythritol 25 drops fluid stevia
- 6 squares unsweetened heating chocolate

DIRECTIONS

1. In a bowl, include avocado, coconut milk, cream and vanilla concentrate. Blend in with an drenching blender until smooth. 2. Include the powdered erythritol, stevia and cocoa powder. Blend well.

3. Break the heating chocolate and fuse to the blend.

4. Spot in the ice chest for 6-12 hours. Expel 20 minutes before serving and include the blend to the dessert machine, adhering to the producer's directions.

NUTRITIONAL INFO PER SERVING

- Calories: 240
- Fat: 22g
- Net Carbs: 4g
- Protein: 4g

CHOCOLATE ROLL CAKE

With a rich chocolate cake and a yummy cream cheddar filling, this cake roll will kick your yearnings to the control in style. SERVES: 12

INGREDIENTS

- For the Mix: 1 cup almond flour 4 tbsp. softened spread 3 eggs ¼ cup psyllium husk powder ¼ cup cocoa powder ¼ cup coconut milk ¼ cup harsh cream ¼ cup erythritol 1 tsp. vanilla 1 tsp. heating powder For the Filling: 8 oz. cream cheddar 8 tbsp. margarine ¼ cup harsh cream ¼ cup erythritol ¼ tsp. stevia 1 tsp. vanilla

DIRECTIONS

1. In a bowl, join all the dry ingredients and gradually include the wet ingredients, blending great.
2. Spread the mixture onto a material paper secured treat sheet. Prepare at 350°F for 12-15 minutes.
3. Make the filling by combining all the ingredients. At the point when the cake is done, spread the filling over it and move cake firmly.

NUTRITION INFO PER SERVING

- Calories: 275
- Fat: 25g
- Net Carbs: 3g
- Protein: 5g

PEANUT BUTTER MILKSHAKE WITH CARAMEL

Nut and caramel flavors consolidate flavorful right now, dessert.

SERVES: 1

INGREDIENTS

- 1 cup coconut milk 7 ice 3D shapes 2 tbsp. nutty spread 2 tbsp. sans sugar salted caramel syrup 1 tbsp. MCT oil ¼ tsp. thickener

DIRECTIONS

1. Include all the ingredients together in a blender, and mix until smooth. Appreciate!

Nourishing INFO PER SERVING

- Calories: 365
- Fat: 35g
- Net Carbs: 5g
- Protein: 8g

MOCHA ICE CREAM

Try not to be tricked into imagining that you can't eat frozen yogurt on a keto diet! Of course, you can! SERVE:S 2

INGREDIENTS

- 1 cup coconut milk
- ¼ cup overwhelming cream
- 2 tbsp. erythritol
- 16 drops fluid stevia

- 2 tbsp. cocoa powder
- 1 tbsp. moment espresso
- ¼ tsp. xanthan gum

DIRECTIONS

1. Include all the ingredients (with the exception of the thickener) into a submersion blender. Mix.
2. Include thickener while mixing. Continue mixing until the blends somewhat thickens.
3. Put in the frozen yogurt machine and adhere to the producer's guidelines.

NUTRITIONAL INFO PER SERVING

- Calories: 146
- Fat: 17g
- Net Carbs: 1.7g
- Protein: 2g

VODKA MOJITO: LOW CARB AND SUGAR

Ingredients

- 4 leaves Mint new
- 2 tbsp Lime Juice 2 Tablespoons
- 2 g Granulated Stevia
- Ice Cubed or Crushed
- 1 shot Vodka
- 1 sprinkle Club Soda
- Lime Slice for Garnish (discretionary)

US Customary - Metric Directions

1. Utilizing a muddler or other utensil, crush new mint leaves with lime and Stevia.
2. Fill glass with ice of inclination. Include vodka.
3. Polish off with club pop.
4. Embellish with a lime cut and mint.
5. Notes
6. 2g net carbs

Nourishment

- Calories: 109kcal | Carbohydrates: 2g | Sodium: 1mg | Vitamin C: 9mg

MAPLE NUT MUFFINS

An incredible treat consolidating maple and walnut, and crammed with fiber!

SERVES 10

INGREDIENTS

- 1 cup almond flour
- ½ cup flaxseed
- ¾ cup walnut (parts)
- ½ cup coconut oil
- 2 eggs
- ¼ cup erythritol
- 2 tsp. maple extricate
- 1 tsp. vanilla concentrate ½ tsp. preparing pop
- ½ tsp. apple juice vinegar ¼ tsp. fluid stevia

DIRECTIONS

1. In a nourishment processor, hack the walnuts. Take ⅓ and put in a safe spot.
2. Consolidate all the wet ingredients in a bowl.
3. Blend the dry ingredients, and include the remainder of the walnuts. Include the wet ingredients and blend well.
4. In a cupcake plate, convey the hitter to make 10 biscuits.
5. Over the top, sprinkle the ⅓ hacked walnuts.
6. Prepare at 325°F for 25-30 minutes.

NUTITRITION INFO PER SERVING

- Calories: 210
- Fat: 20g
- Net Carbs: 1.6g

KETO BOMBS

Consolidate chocolate and nutty spread, and give yourself a merited treat in twofold fast time! SERVES: 2

INGREDIENTS

- 2 tbsp. nutty spread 1 tbsp. substantial cream 1 tbsp. coconut oil 1 tsp. cocoa powder ¼ tsp. allspice Fluid sucralose

DIRECTIONS

1. Into a cup or form, put the nutty spread, include the coconut oil, substantial cream, cocoa powder and allspice. Blend well.
2. Freeze for two hours and expel.

NUTRITION INFO PER SERVING

- Calories: 385
- Fat: 40g
- Net Carbs: 8g
- Protein: 8g

CARAMEL FAT BOMBS

Planning time: 5 minutes Cooking time: 0 minutes Serves: 36

INGREDIENTS:

- 1 cup spread, relaxed to room temperature
- 1 cup coconut oil
- ¼ cup sharp cream

- ¼ cup overwhelming whipping cream
- Caramel sugar and sugar to taste
- Coarse ground ocean salt

DIRECTIONS:

1. Consolidate the margarine and coconut oil in a blending bowl and blend well.
2. Include the sharp cream, substantial cream, caramel sugar, and sugar and blend well in with a rush until very much joined.
3. Empty the blend into molds, sprinkle with ocean salt and spot in the cooler.
4. At the point when the fat bombs become strong, expel from the shape and appreciate.
5. Store them in the refrigerator.

NOURISHMENT FACTS (PER SERVING)

- Total Carbohydrates: 0g Dietary
- Fiber: 0g
- Net Cabs: 0g
- Protein: 0g
- Complete Fat: 12g
- Calories: 100

COCONUT CINNAMON FAT BOMBS

Planning time: 5 minutes Cooking time: 0 minutes Serves: 6

INGREDIENTS:

- 4 tablespoons spread, relaxed
- 4 ounces cream cheddar
- 2 tablespoons additional virgin coconut oil

- Run of cinnamon
- Sprinkle of vanilla concentrate
- 2 Splenda parcels or without sugar of your decision, to taste

DIRECTIONS:

1. In a little bowl, join the spread, cream cheddar, and coconut oil.
2. Include the sugar, cinnamon and vanilla. Blend well until the blend gets smooth.
3. Spoon the blend into a treat form (any shape) or ice 3D shape plate and place in the cooler for 3-4 hours.
4. Pop the confections out and appreciate.

NUTRITION FACTS (PER SERVING)

- Total Carbohydrates: 1 g Dietary
- Fiber: 0g
- Net Cabs: 0g
- Protein: 1g
- All out Fat: 18g
- Calories: 165

SIMPLE KETO BROWNIE

Only 3 minutes and you can have this yummy chocolaty dessert in your face!

SERVES 1

INGREDIENTS

- 2 eggs 1 tbsp. granulated sugar 1 scoop protein powder 1 tbsp. overwhelming cream

DIRECTIONS

1. In a mug, include the eggs, overwhelming cream, granulated sugar and protein powder. Blend well.
2. Microwave for 1 moment.

Dietary INFO PER SERVING

*   Calories: 310
*   Fat: 15g
*   Net Carbs: 5g
*   Protein: 35g

LOW-CARB COOKIES

An exemplary transformed into this solid choice for you and the children. Make them as a family movement! SERVES 18

INGREDIENTS

*   2½ cups whitened almond flour ¼ cup shelled and slashed pecans ½ cup unsalted margarine 2 eggs ½ cup powdered erythritol ½ cup dim chocolate chips Salt ½ tsp. heating soft drink 1 tbsp. vanilla concentrate

DIRECTIONS

1. In a bowl, join almond flour, salt, preparing pop and erythritol.
2. Independently, blend softened spread and vanilla, chocolate chips, eggs and pecans. Join with the dry blend until you have batter.
3. Make treats with 1 scoop of the mixture per treat and spot them onto a treat sheet. 4. Heat for 8-10 at 350°F. Cool for 10 minutes.

NOURISHING INFO PER SERVING

- Calories: 172
- Fat: 15g
- Net Carbs: 3g
- Protein: 0g

MICROWAVE BROWNIE

For occupied individuals who need a brownie dessert, this formula will turn into a go-to for at the point when you're lacking in time. SERVES 1

INGREDIENTS

- 1 tbsp. smooth almond margarine, 1 tbsp. beaten egg white, 1 tsp. unsweetened cocoa powder ⅛ tsp. vanilla concentrate 3 drops fluid sucralose or on the other hand stevia Baking pop Salt, Almonds or walnuts, orange or lemon extricate (discretionary)

DIRECTIONS

1. Beat egg whites in a bowl until they are foamy.
2. In a microwave-safe cup, blend the egg white blend with the remainder of the ingredients.
3. Microwave for 40 seconds and expel.

NUTRITION INFO PER SERVING

- Calories: 105
- Fat: 9g
- Net Carbs: 3g

CHOCOLATE COOKIES

Is it evident we love treats? With practically 15g carbs and 20g protein per serving, it's anything but difficult to perceive any reason why.

SERVES 16

INGREDIENTS

- 7 tbsp. spread, 2 cups almond flour, ¾ cup granulated sugar 2 oz. dull chocolate 2 eggs, 1 tbsp. orange get-up-and-go, 1 tbsp. squeezed orange 1 tsp. orange concentrate 1 tsp. vanilla concentrate ¾ tsp. preparing, powder ½ tsp. preparing soft drink ½ tsp. salt

DIRECTIONS

1. Blend the almond flour, preparing pop, heating powder, salt, and granulated sugar.
2. Dissolve the spread in a microwave-safe bowl and afterward blend it in with the orange juice, orange get-up-and-go, orange concentrate and vanilla concentrate.
3. Consolidate the two blends and include the split up chocolate and eggs. Ensure they are all around blended.
4. Spot the batter broiler a heating sheet on a treat sheet, shaping square shapes and cut it into 16.
5. Prepare at 350°F for around 20-25 minutes.

NUTRITION INFO PER SERVING

- Calories: 155
- Fat: 14g
- Net Carbs: 10g
- Protein: 17g

LOW CARB SHORTBREAD

The lemon and rosemary right now shortbread improve things greatly. Make a group and offer them out with loved ones. SERVES 24

INGREDIENTS

- 2 cups almond flour
- ½ tsp. heating pop
- ½ tsp. heating powder
- ⅓ cup granulated sugar
- 6 tbsp. margarine
- 1 tsp. vanilla concentrate
- 1 tbsp. lemon pizzazz, ground 4 tsp. lemon juice
- 2 tsp. rosemary, dried or new

DIRECTIONS

1. In a bowl, join almond flour, preparing powder, heating pop and sugar.
2. Liquefy the spread in a microwave, and include the vanilla concentrate, lemon pizzazz, lemon juice and rosemary. Consolidate the dried blend mixing gradually. At the point when done, envelop the batter by a saran wrap and spot in the cooler for 30 minutes.
3. Expel the mixture from the cooler, and cut it into 12 pieces.
4. Heat for 15 minutes at 350°F on a lubed treat sheet with salted spread.

At the point when done, let cool for 10 minutes.

NOURISHING INFO PER SERVING

- Calories: 80

- Fat: 7g
- Net Carbs: 1g
- Protein: 2g